ISBN 0 9511868 0 9

Prepared for publication by
Jenny Lee Publishing Services
Bishop's Stortford, Herts
Phototypeset by Wyvern Typesetting Ltd, Bristol
Printed in Great Britain by J. W. Arrowsmith Ltd, Bristol

*I would like to give thanks to my son
Jonathan for all the artwork
contained in this book.*

Write for details of courses to:

Ann Gillanders,
The Holistic Healing Centre,
92 Sheering Road,
Old Harlow,
Essex, CM17 0JT

Tel. Harlow (0279) 29060

# Reflexolog

*The ancient answer
to modern ailments*

**Ann Gillanders**

# Contents

# List of figures

# Introduction

Allow me to introduce you to the subject of foot reflexology. Often referred to as compression massage of the feet, it is a natural and drugless way of healing the body by using its own natural healing resources. Like acupuncture, reflexology has been used in China for 5,000 years. In A.D. 1027 it is recorded as having been used as an energy-balancing procedure.

In the last twenty years reflexology has been making a slow but sure impact in the field of alternative therapies and today proves to be a very safe and effective way of stimulating all functions, organs and other parts of the body by means of pressure to small areas in the feet called 'reflex points'. These areas are only the size of pinheads, so the accuracy of the therapist in detecting these areas and working on them is of paramount importance. No gadgets or 'aids' are necessary; in fact, I feel that the greatest 'sin' one can commit is to use probes or electrical stimulating devices. You only need two hands which can be trained to work in a very specific, controlled way. Hands were meant for healing, but in order to become a proficient therapist you need to have a genuine compassion for the suffering of mankind, a good basic knowledge of the working of the human body and the acceptance that you cannot become a reflexologist overnight. You must also accept that it takes time to get a result from treatment sessions just as it took some time to become ill. All too frequently I find that people expect an instant miracle at their first appointment.

I have tried to change the content of this book on reflexology, which perhaps makes it different from any others. My aim has been to whet the appetite of those interested in exploring the field of alternative medicine with the renewed interest of today's world and to concentrate upon researching into the historical background of holistic medicine which gave rise to reflexology.

We should also understand that the term 'alternative medicine' is far from accurate. Natural medicines were used from the very beginning of time. The orthodox and conventional forms of treatment are really very recent, so surely *they* should be referred to as 'alternative'! Care in health and sickness are becoming the responsibility of the individual. I have been treating sick and suffering people for many years and have found that reflexology is one of the best and most effective ways of helping people to help themselves.

Just as matter evolves, so does man's knowledge. Through actual practice our knowledge is continuously developed and increased, making this therapy an even more effective method for the prevention and relief of disease.

I have developed and grown spiritually as the result of my work and I would like to share with you what I have learnt through theoretical study, practical experience and much historical research.

# 1 Man and nature

Although all healing was intended to be simple in its origin, through the ages man has tried to change it. Herbalism is one of the most ancient forms of medicine, but man has largely destroyed the herbs, roots and shrubs which are available and which have been poisoned by chemical sprays. These were provided to help man find some relief from his health problems. Not only have we destroyed the herbs, roots and shrubs but we have also polluted our air with diesel and petrol fumes, waste discharged from industrial factories, and the powerful chemicals that are used on our fields. Moreover, we even have chemicals in our drinking water. So as we eat vegetables that are grown in polluted soil, breathe air that is full of fumes and drink water that is not pure, it is hardly surprising that the health of our nation is in a chronic state. When we load all these destructive elements together and lace them with high-powered living, tension, worry, frustration and the fight to possess more and more material goods, it is difficult to imagine how mankind survives at all.

Nature opened the very first drugstore. Primitive man and animals depended on preventive use of its stock of plants and herbs to avoid disease and to maintain health and strength. Because man and animals were constantly on the move, nature's drugstore had branches everywhere. Wherever in the world you were sick you would find in the fields its medicines to cure you (and I mean 'cure', not 'suppress', which has nothing whatsoever to do with healing). Primitive man used infusions of herbs to take internally and ointments for skin complaints.

Our pioneering ancestors discovered the principles of healing by observing how the animals cured themselves from disease. I have come to marvel at the instinct of animals to make use of natural laws to heal themselves. They know exactly what herbs will cure specific ills. Wild creatures first seek solitude and absolute relaxation, then they rely on the complete remedies of nature, the medicine in plants and pure air. An animal with a fever quickly hunts up an airy, shady place near water, there remaining quiet, eating nothing and drinking frequently until its health is recovered. On the other hand, an animal disabled by rheumatism finds a spot in hot sunlight and lies in it until the pain almost bakes out of its system. However, man, in a sense, tends to be a rebel against nature and a deserter from the animal kingdom.

Take an animal's refusal to eat when it is sick. By letting food alone it creates within its body a new biochemical state which assists in hastening recovery. Humans have a habit of feeling that if they miss a meal something terrible will happen to them. They do not remember that the body stores reserves against time of need and could maintain itself, if necessary, without taking any food at all, for the length of time of the average illness.

Turning to the subject of exercise, we can study the animals too and note what they do. First of all they roam the fields in search of food, which means that they walk a great deal. A young animal is extremely active: puppies and kittens are forever on the go, running, climbing and exploring. With the passing years body activity is directed towards securing food and defending itself and its offspring against enemy attack. If we would take a leaf out of the animal book, we would exercise more. Leisure time in the animal kingdom is spent resting the body so that it will be ready to seek food or fight to defend itself.

With the changing seasons, when their systems require certain adjustments, unerring instinct causes animals to change their diet. When they are on their own none of the foods they find is refined. They are not finicky, and they accept food in a natural state as nature prepared it for them.

It is sometimes very difficult to grasp that once we were microscopic specks. Oliver Wendell Holmes used to say that the life of the individual begins a hundred years before he is born. It is certain that we do not start physiologically at birth but nine months before coming into the world. The speck which is our beginning becomes alive through foods. It takes shelter, steady temperature, elimination of waste and a healthy mother to give an infant a good start.

If one hopes to be a successful gardener one soon learns in the garden the necessity of reinforcing soil with nitrogen, phosphorus and potassium. The nitrogen is for leaf growth, the phosphorus is to produce flowers, and potassium is for strength of root and stem. If any of these elements are left out the plant will suffer.

Honey was regarded as a medicine and used extensively. It prevents gastro-intestinal fermentation which leads to many disorders of the bowel. It contains an important element for forming new blood and, having a mild laxative effect, it prevents constipation. Being also a body sedative it helps promote sound sleep and, if given to infants, helps build a good nervous system.

I feel that what is missing in the conventional approach to health today is 'touch'. Most aches and pains are treated by doctors with bottles of pills, and I think I am right in saying that it is on infrequent occasions that doctors examine patients and achieve any contact. The treatment of disease is mechanical. We have equipment that looks terrifying, monitoring devices, all forms of X-ray, radiotherapy and chemotherapy, all of which must create much fear in the patient, and a very cold, clinical approach to suffering.

Doctors of old had little aid to offer their patients; there were few drugs, mild pain-killing tablets, bottles of cough medicine, laxatives and various 'rub-in' oils for painful joints or muscle sprains. I understand that a very effective and much-used remedy for painful joints or muscle sprains was 'horse-oils'! This was a concoction of wintergreen, camphor, juniper and liquid paraffin. It was used originally to help lame horses. However, doctors used to be with their patients during a 'healing crisis', particularly in cases of pneumonia, bronchitis and rheumatic fever, and most doctors were assessed on their bedside manner.

Disease is an integral part of the human condition. There is no possible way we can eliminate it from our lives. Humankind evolves through health and sickness. We learn from both. We see sickness as bad, so we attack it by means of powerful and often harmful drugs. Any hint of discomfort calls for an immediate visit to the doctor for a prescription. Most often doctors and drugs serve only to make illness less painful. The body has its own way of coping with physical imbalance, and drugs often prolong or interfere with the body's healing process. Modern medicine is preoccupied with getting rid of or masking symptoms, and this may be the major reason why it is so ineffective.

The holistic health philosophy considers the body as a dynamic energy system which is in a constant state of change. Human beings are more than just their bodies. Each is a complex balance of mental, physical and spiritual aspects that are integrated into and affected directly by environmental and social factors. The cause of illness is far more deep-rooted than external symptoms. We live in an age of scientific specialization; each part of the body is viewed and treated as separate from the rest.

We are all deceivers to one degree or another – if not verbally, then emotionally. What do you do when you feel an emotion while relating to another person, but would rather not have that person observe your reaction? Most people hold back emotion by tensing muscles, in a way subtle enough that your friend will be unaware of the tension. Nevertheless, that tension does exist and becomes buried away as an almost unconscious fear.

Sometimes we have an unconscious fear of expressing our emotions in a natural way, a conditioned response carried over from early childhood. Let your mind wander into the past and try to remember how very natural, healthy emotional outbursts were handled by your parents. If your family was like mine and most others, I would guess that natural outbursts that your parents saw as inappropriate were swiftly suppressed with a slap, a cold stare, a threat or – most effective of all – a withdrawal of love. All children are subject to conditioning, just as Pavlov conditioned dogs. Rewards are given for responses deemed appropriate by those in control, not necessarily for natural responses. Repression of emotions results from voluntary suppression that has become unconscious habit. It should be apparent that each response to stress involves an increase in bodily tension. Emotions are actually stored in the body in the form of chronic muscle tension and are a primary cause of headaches, back pain and poor posture. Common slang such as 'uptight' is often very accurate and perceptive. If we repress emotions we get uptight, our muscles tense and the natural flow of energy in our bodies is obstructed.

Emotions are like rivers: there are rapids and areas of calm flowing waters, there are unpredictable bends, and the course of the river is likely to change many times throughout its lifetime. If the flow is obstructed by a dam it does not stop the flow completely; water still rushes in. The water backs up, floods the surrounding countryside and forms a reservoir which also needs to be controlled. If the water is not controlled it might burst the dam, and then such a release will cause far more damage to the countryside than if the river had been unimpeded by a dam. Emotions, like rivers, need unobstructed flow and your restraint will not make them go away.

Sometimes illness is a built-in defence mechanism that helps you avoid life situations that you just cannot face. Sometimes it is a way of enforcing a stop when you have been working overtime for a ridiculously long period or perhaps you are trying to establish a new business and feel guilty about having any time off; so illness makes the decision for you. Illness can be a way of creating some love and attention if you have been feeling neglected by your spouse and children, or it can be a way of making you more sympathetic to the real suffering of others. Perhaps you have been selfish or even cruel for too long with little thought for the rest of the world; sickness can then teach you to be more understanding. Sickness enables you to be excused from many decision-making situations; little will be expected of you if most of the time you are unwell.

I have treated many very unhappily married women in my years as a reflexologist. They all present with a chronic health state, allergies, migraine and bowel troubles and very frequently back pain, plus episodes of 'depression'. They are full of frustrations and bitterness, and complain about the wasted years with their partner. When you ask, 'Why do you stay and put up with the situation if things are so bad?' the answer is usually that there would be no one to cut the grass, tend to the repairs, run the car and so on, and then of course, 'There is my migraine, I could not possibly hold down a job'. The migraine is a convenient escape from making a decision to end their unhappy state, to have to stand on their own feet, earn a living and be responsible for their own future.

I remember a friend of mine whom I treated for migraine. She was very unhappy in a disastrous marriage. She started to make an excellent recovery after only a very few treatments, her attacks became fewer and fewer and she obviously saw good health for the future and immediately stopped having treatment. That was also the end of our so-called 'friendship', as she never spoke to me again. It is very sad when you see so many people who do not want to 'lose their illness'.

I knew a man who was full of self, he was often verbally cruel, domineering and very overbearing. He was full of ego and proud of his so-called 'health and strength'. One day disaster struck and he lost a leg in a train crash and eventually recovered sufficiently to be fitted for an artificial limb which he mastered well. What a change came over that man. He was in a large ward full of patients who had undergone major surgery, many had lost a limb or limbs. He watched the suffering and uncomplaining attitude of little children as they struggled to gain mobility with artificial limbs, and as he said to me, 'My whole selfish rotten life flashed before my eyes', and he realized just what he was and also the misery he had caused to so many people. What had he of any real importance? – 'nothing'. His wife had left him years before and, as he said, 'She was justified'. His children had lost contact with him, and somewhere out there he knew that he had grandchildren whom he had never seen.

Not only did he have to suffer the pain of losing a limb but he had to go through the intense emotional pain of 'loneliness' as he lay in that hospital ward watching all the 'love' that came through those doors for other people. The visitors, the flowers, the cards and the care. Nobody came to visit him, he had given no love and so there was no 'return' for him.

What a change came over that man! He had been a very clever engineer and eventually founded a factory for the development and construction of light-weight 'cosmetic' limbs and calipers, a great step forward from the ugly steel and leather contraptions of the past. The rest of his life served a useful purpose, being involved with people who needed his expertise. As his factory became larger and larger he funded a home for disabled children. Unfortunately he had to lose a limb to 'grow' spiritually and develop his neglected talent.

# 2  Chinese teachings and healing

In China there is a strong movement amongst medical practitioners to mine the treasures of traditional Chinese medicine – acupuncture, herbal medicine, reflexology and massage – and to combine these with the best of Western medicine. With the ever-increasing awareness of the risks or dangerous side effects as well as the costs accompanying the use of many Western drug therapies, Chinese medicine is rapidly growing. Thousands of years ago the Chinese doctor only received payment for his treatment when the patient was well. Even if a very elderly patient died the doctor received nothing, and was considered ultimately responsible for his failure in restoring the patient to health.

Reflexology is a form of 'holistic healing'. The term 'holistic' is taken from the Greek word 'holos', meaning whole, and in accordance with any holistic principle three aspects must be involved in order to achieve a feeling of well-being – the mind, the body and the spirit.

Ancient Chinese philosophy regarded the human organism as a miniature version of the universe and often referred to man as 'the small world'. According to the Chinese concept the processes which occur within the human organism, including illnesses, are connected with the interplay of the five elements which I will explore in more detail later in this chapter. Man cannot therefore be divorced from nature; he forms an organic part of it and is closely linked to the universe. Therefore nature as a macrocosm and man as a microcosm obey much the same laws.

The head was associated with the firmament, the hair with the stars and constellations, the eyes and ears with the sun and the moon. Human breath – the soul – corresponded to the wind (the Greek word for wind was 'pneuma', from which the word 'pneumonia' came). Blood was equated with rain, while the blood vessels were streams and rivers. The remaining functions and structures were classified as follows.

The human body corresponded to earth itself; the skeleton represented the mountains; the heart was the constellation of the Great Bear; while the five elements – wood, fire, earth, metal and water – corresponded to the five internal organs, the lungs, heart, kidneys, spleen and liver. The four seasons had a significance too, as they were said to correspond to the four limbs, and the twelve months to the twelve large sections of the body. The very primitive cosmic magical view is also reflected in the concept in which the sky corresponded to the head and the earth to the stomach.

There was a school in China which compared the body to the state. Dr Ko Hung, who lived in the first half of the fourth century B.C., compared in his manuscript the thorax and abdominal region to the palaces and courts, the limbs to the frontiers, the bones and joints to the various classes of officials, the spirit to the ruler, the blood to the ministers, but energy (which keeps the whole body alive) to the people. The fact that this concept, if not in the medical sense, had a basic truth and meaning becomes evident from the conclusion he drew. 'The people provide life. If the people are fed the state can endure. If not then the state too perishes.' Man must therefore obey the laws of the universe.

We shall now devote our attention to the doctrine of the five elements which have a strong relativity in the teachings of life itself as well as a strong basis in Chinese philosophies and cultures. The five elements are wood, earth, metal, water and fire. They can exist in a helpful and complementary relationship to one another or they can work against one another and so destroy themselves. The doctrine of the elements has its origins in very ancient concepts.

It is perhaps possible to interpret it in the following way. Fire is fed by wood. After the fire has burned itself out there remains ashes which become earth, in which metals are found and from which water springs. The water feeds the trees and this completes the circle back to the element of wood. Such a sequence is, in part, supported by the traditional art of healing.

The mind fuels the body with negative or positive thoughts.

11

Negative thoughts breed destructive elements. Destructive elements create tension and constriction of circulation. Disease manifests in tense, sluggish areas of the body. The organs become diseased and fail to function. Our thinking becomes even more disturbed and negative, pain permeates most of our days, which causes us to become more and more dissociated from nature. Our vital energy becomes weaker and weaker, we die and go back to the earth.

The traditional art of healing stressed the importance of investigating climatic influences in connection with various illnesses. Ever since ancient times it has been observed that climate, seasons and variations in temperature, on the one hand, and a balanced state of bodily health, on the other, were related. Spring is the season of increasing vitality, a time of restitution. During the summer months there is evidence of an increase in cardiac disease and 'intermittent fever' (malaria). In autumn the forces between heaven and earth balance out, and this season can be harmful for the lungs. Finally, winter is the period when nature rests and it is now that kidney diseases frequently occur. It was also noted that windy weather in spring caused diarrhoea and that summer heat brought on feverish illness. The autumnal dampness coincided with coughing and the winter cold with feverish ailments, particularly childhood illnesses which broke out in spring.

In the fourth century B.C. Dr Ko Hung stated in his manuscript on man and nature, 'If man eats too many salt things his veins will become stiff and the colour of his skin will change.' We know today that salt has a detrimental effect on the arteries, is greatly responsible for arteriosclerosis and indeed does cause the skin to change colour. As the arteries become corroded blood is restricted, in particular, to the lower limbs, giving the legs a clay-like appearance.

He also wrote, 'If man eats too much sweet food his bones will be painful.' We know today that the excessive quantities of sugar in our diet since the war years is responsible for the increase in the rheumatic and arthritic conditions of joints.

He also wrote of an 'acid mind' causing an acid body and writes that 'an evil and black thinking mind will eventually invade the body's defences and cause black corrosions within'. In order to 'whiten' the body the mind must first be cleansed. It is interesting to me to note that way back in the fourth century B.C. it was accepted that the mind had a dramatic effect on the body. Today we are just beginning to accept this fact!

At the beginning of the seventh century B.C. the first medical training school was set up in China by imperial decree. According to tradition some three hundred doctors are said to have studied at this school, and there were some outstanding teachers who instructed in acupuncture, remedial massage and 'magic spells'. The latter were introduced into the art of healing through Buddhist influence, but they never played an important part.

The general art of healing at this time concerned itself with surgery, the curing of children's ailments, moxibustion and cupping. This is a very painful treatment where heated 'cups' are placed over the part of the body that is painful, in an attempt to draw out the toxicity. Whether or not this was successful is difficult to say, but it did cause quite excessive burns to the area treated. Also treated were diseases of the eyes, nose and ears, and dentistry was performed. Success in treatment was believed to correspond to simplicity and application.

In A.D. 1017 Dr Wang Wei had a human figure cast in bronze on which were marked those points on the body important for acupuncture. The students practised on this bronze figure in locating these parts on the body.

When this knowledge was put into practice in treating the sick, practitioners positioned the needles in the appropriate areas of the body and then applied deep pressure therapy on the soles of the inside and outside edge of both feet. They then applied a concentrated pressure on the big toe. The reason they used the feet in conjunction with the acupuncture needles was to channel extra energy through the body. Dr Wang Wei said that the feet were the most sensitive parts of all and contained great energizing areas.

I feel sure that they were working upon the reflex to the pituitary gland, which is found in the big toe. They then worked upon the reflex to the solar plexus, which is found at the bases of the metatarsals. Working on the inside of both feet would be contacting the reflex points to the entire spine and on the outside edge of the feet we would find the reflexes to the hip and pelvic areas. These five areas are usually the most sensitive in 95 per cent of people.

If we compare from a chronological point of view the treasures of the Chinese art of healing and the great historical personalities of Chinese medicine with the important figures and events in the history of Western medicine, it will be seen that Pien Chueh, 'the father of the pulse', was probably a contemporary of the Greek physician Hippocrates, the father of Western medicine (*c*.460–*c*.370 B.C.). Diagnosis by means of taking the pulse (a tradition in China which is 2,500 years old), anaesthesia as early as the second century B.C. and the first use of a primitive form of vaccine, all show that in many respects the Chinese art of healing was well in advance of its Western counterpart. Skulls found during excavations further reveal that cranial operations were practised in China thousands of years ago.

It is therefore very difficult to accept the subsequent progress of modern Western medicine and the ensuing stagnation of the traditional Chinese arts of healing. To understand this situation it is necessary to have a clear picture of the social and historical developments in China.

Many people believed that the traditional Chinese art of healing was composed of some mysterious and magical knowledge which derived from a long dead 'golden era' and which far exceeds modern medicine in value, but this view is not correct. Chinese medicine, as Western medicine, was also hindered in its development.

The first healers or medicine men were a type of shaman who understood more about the healing of injuries and skin diseases than they did about the treatment of internal ailments. They also used magic spells in which the rational and mystical elements have been confused. The evidence of oracle bones suggests that the main body of knowledge at the beginning of the antique period concerned abdominal injuries, diseases of the ear, nose, eye, mouth and teeth, and bone fractures. Stone needles were used for the opening of boils and abscesses, and the principle of cranial surgery was also understood.

During the Ming period (A.D. 1368–1644), after the Mongols had been driven out, there was a great upsurge in trade, which in turn strengthened the power of the towns. Towards the end of the Ming dynasty Europe was entering an age of discoveries, European navigators brought back spices and drugs, and so it was that camphor arrived from China together with opium, which was originally used in that country as a medicine.

During this progressive period more than fifty medical works were published in China on the subject of smallpox, and about the middle of the sixteenth century it was discovered that the secretion from smallpox vesicles or dried vesicles themselves in powdered form were a powerful means of immunization. The powder was sniffed into the nose. This method of immunization, which had long been used in popular medicine, was also adopted by Russian doctors who transmitted it to Turkey. As far as the West was concerned it was not until 1796 that immunization against smallpox was discovered by an Englishman, Edward Jenner. So back we must go, to the beginning of time, to understand the development of natural medicine, to understand the Chinese philosophies, the use of acupuncture, reflexology and all forms of 'touch therapies'.

How, you will ask, does applying pressure to sensitive vital areas in the feet relieve pain and suffering? It is generally considered that pressure therapy – which is indeed reflexology – has the ability to flush out the tissues and improve the circulation of the blood and accordingly make the joints more flexible. I feel that it has a reflective effect on nerve functions, causing the excitory process of the nervous system to reach an equilibrium of balance, and this, in turn, produces a medical effect. Many books written on the subject of reflexology refer to 'crystalline deposits in the feet' which cause the pain. I find this a disturbing and inexplicable statement. What I do believe is that the disorder in the physical body causes a reflex action in the feet and triggers the 'pain zone' as a reflex in the extremity, which is the feet. For example, if a patient suffers from sciatica, he or she may have limited pain in the hip area but extreme pain

15

radiating from knee to ankle. Therefore, the inflammation in the sciatic nerve caused a reflective reaction on the 'zone' throughout the body. Pressure therefore on the reflex area in the foot will be sensitive, signalling the state of an organ, gland, function or part in that zone.

If a patient suffers from an inflammatory condition of a nerve in the neck, he/she may suffer limited discomfort in the neck but have great pain in the fingers. We also hear mention medically of 'referred pain'; this gives a similar explanation. We must always therefore compare the human body to the elements of nature. The largest and mightiest oak tree relies on drawing on the earth and receiving its life-giving sustenance, and water, minerals and carbon dioxide from the air which it changes into sugars. The most beautiful flower cannot survive if its stem becomes weakened in any way. Even if you prop it up with a thin stick, and even if the stem is only damaged and not severed, the bloom will rapidly become very dejected, wither away and die. I feel that disease manifests itself when there is a 'kink' or imbalance in the zonal pathways of the body.

Through the wonderful healing principles that reflexology offers we can rechannel this energy through the body. Let us now accept that our feet need to be 'in tune' with the rest of our body, that our body draws on an energy from the ground which we receive through our feet. Today we need manual stimulation of the soles of our feet to help our bodies, but years ago when man walked the earth with bare feet he received this stimulating life force every day of his life.

# 3 Reflexology and the medical profession

Reflexology is a practical science, a simple science and a safe one, as the only instrument we need to master the art are just two hands!

In physical medicine methods are used to try to alleviate pain and discomfort. We, as reflexologists, do the same by relaxing the patient and relieving nervous tension. It is my belief that reflexology should be part of every physical medicine department in hospitals, as its use as a diagnostic tool is infallible.

It is most unfortunate that many a physician in the field of medicine will try to remove from competition anyone who helps people to get well, unless of course that individual is another medical practitioner. Unless a physician is basically insecure, no one should pose a threat to him. In fact, I understand that the death rate of physicians from coronary heart disease is on the increase, so these people should welcome our assistance as we must lighten their load.

It has been assessed that doctors who show little personal interest in their patients are seldom liked by them, and their placebo power is diminished. Not only do the personality and attitude of the doctor affect the success of a treatment, but so also does the attitude and personality of the patient alter the course of disease. A positive mental attitude has been shown to improve the chances of survival for women with breast cancer.

People decide when to be ill. It has been found that 90 per cent of the population experience some symptoms of illness in any two-week period, with an average of four symptoms each. Ulcers, asthma, high blood pressure, backache and angina are all nowadays acknowledged to have a strong psychological background, and there is increasing evidence of a mental factor in the development of cancer.

It is medically accepted that 75 per cent of all disease is caused by stress. The greatest benefit one can receive from reflexology is relaxation, so we must surely be well on the way to helping so many sick and suffering people, and the wonderful thing about this natural way to restore health is that it is far superior to drugs which, years later, leave their marks. No mind should ever be closed so far as patient care is concerned. The main objective in healing should be to help the sick person regardless of the type of medical help which was sought. The practitioner should in no way feel 'threatened' or 'insulted' because a patient received his benefit through some form of holistic healing.

Doctors are trained to work on human beings as if they were mechanics repairing parts of a motor car that was broken down, a method that is highly effective when treating accident victims but somewhat lacking when it comes to acute and chronic disease.

It is not difficult to see how illness can be created by mood and feelings. The hormonal system controlled by the pituitary gland in the brain is very responsive to changes in mood. The adrenal/pituitary glands are sensitive to any external stressful events. The mental control over involuntary organs and the control of the nervous system with biofeedback machines also demonstrates the great ability of the mind to control disease in the body. Blood pressure can be lowered, and a whole host of conditions from migraine to muscle paralysis and asthma can be improved by mental willpower and a biofeedback machine.

If you have benefited from a series of reflexology sessions, tell your doctor about your experience – he may give it some serious thought. Doctors learn from their patients; that is how they got where they are today, by taking detailed histories, doing physical examinations and collating information. The theory they received in the classroom; the rest was learnt by caring for patients.

I hope I live to see the day when medical doctors, osteopaths, herbalists, reflexologists, chiropractors and homeopaths will all work together with one goal in mind, preventive health care. I would also like to see the government providing funds to educate the young in how to prevent their bodies becoming ill, instead of pouring millions into the production of ever more new drugs which promise us 'the answer to disease'; then frequently within months of these drugs being marketed they are removed from sale because of serious side effects!

I would like natural health sciences to be taught in our schools as an interesting science subject, and the young taught about a natural diet and vegetarianism, about the dangers of the chemicals that are used in our food production. And what about learning total mental and physical relaxation techniques? Unless we are offered and taught about alternatives how can we ever have the freedom to choose the way we want our bodies treated when they are sick. What normally happens is that mankind seeks out alternative therapies when all else has failed and then regrets the years of suffering which he could have avoided.

It is very true when we say 'the more we know about life, the more we worry'. With the development of radio, television, travel and newspapers we are kept up to date hourly with the problems of the world. In the past, many people lived in small communes or villages, and life was simple and uncomplicated, people heard nothing of what was going on fifty miles away, let alone 5,000. It was normal to be born and die in the same village, to farm and live off the land. The women kept house and gave birth to many children, several of whom were destined to die in the first year. There was a lot of physical heavy hard work, but very little tension. The main problem was 'weather conditions'. It was either too wet to harvest, or not wet enough to make the crops grow. The needs of families were simple. The sons and daughters married and lived in the same village, or one very nearby, and repeated the same routine as their parents. Women were old at fifty, but in effect their ignorance of the world situation was 'bliss'. They were not subjected to the threat of nuclear war, over-population, AIDS and other sexually transmitted diseases, or the constant pathetic sights of the starving millions whose disease-wracked bodies are presented to us via our television screens. There was not the constant violence, murder, rape and other atrocities that we have to contend with today.

The body was not built to receive toxins of any kind, and every drug that is taken has a destructive effect on yet another function of the human body. Drugs suppress disease and suppression has nothing to do with healing. They ease pain and relieve symptoms but they do not put right that which caused the body to become sick in the first place.

I am not condemning the use of drugs at all costs. In road accidents, when morphia is available to ease terrible pain, that is indeed a 'wonder drug', and if you have an acute bout of pneumonia then penicillin will do wonders and modern anaesthetics are safe and effective, but I am against the use and abuse of drugs for every ache, pain, mood or sniffle.

Western medicine has explored and technologically refined four areas of treating disease: diagnosis, medicines, chemotherapy and surgery. It has done comparatively little to improve the overall health of the population and to find the true cause of illnesses so that they can be dealt with effectively. We have been brainwashed to believe that illness is caused by germs or viruses that suddenly attack us without cause or provocation and make us ill. This does not mean that doctors think all disease is caused by germs. When illness is not attributed to invasion of the body by micro-organisms, diseases such as cancer, heart disease and multiple sclerosis as well as the large range of demyelinating illnesses which are on the increase are labelled 'cause unknown'.

Each of us carries the potential to contract any disease at any time. However, only certain people do actually become ill where others stay healthy. It is well known that at a certain pharmaceutical laboratory volunteers are invited to the laboratory as human guinea pigs, and the common cold virus is dropped into their noses and throats daily in an attempt to induce an infection. Only one-third of those volunteers will develop an infection; the others fail to respond, no matter how large a dose of live virus they are subjected to. Research completed at the Cold Research Laboratory in 1979 shows also that colds are most likely to strike individuals who are introverted and who have allowed the stresses of life to interfere with their social life and their work.

I firmly believe that the mental and physical condition of the body causes subtle changes in the hormonal and defence mechanisms, thereby allowing the disease or virus to get a hold or to manifest. If the conditions are right, therefore, disease will flourish. Rather like the growth process of the common mushroom, it adores dark damp cold surroundings and will grow in profusion in these conditions; but expose it to sunlight and it will quickly die.

Medicine is at a crossroads today. Developments in the fields of psychiatry, hypnosis and holistic care, coupled with explorations into the nature of consciousness, give convincing evidence that we, as individuals, cause most, if not all, of our own health problems.

Sufferers from allergic illness, hay fever, eczema, asthma and varying types of skin diseases are always treated by the medical profession by drugs to suppress the asthma or hay fever and steroid-based creams to apply to the skin. All illness is caused from problems within manifesting on the outside. Symptoms, whether they be itching, sneezing or scratching, are evidence of an internal build-up of irritation which expresses itself in the symptoms described.

Many asthmatic sufferers will agree that when the asthma is in a virulent stage, their associated eczema will disappear or at least be much improved. When the eczema is at its worst, the asthma is usually at its best, which proves that you cannot suppress nature. If you suppress one part, another area will become diseased.

We talk of these allergic illnesses as of nervous origin. I agree that most sufferers from allergic illnesses present as very sensitive, intense individuals. Their sensitivity may well 'trigger' an outbreak or attack, but the cause still comes from within. To become sensitive to external irritants – such as grass pollen, house dust, animal fur, roses or spring flowers – the body's defence mechanism must be defective. What we need to do is not to treat the allergy but to find out why the body became allergic. Many people who have an acute allergic reaction to pollens and grass find that suddenly their allergy disappears for several years, or permanently. The grasses and pollens are still in abundance, but that person's defences were able, at that time, to cope with the situation.

The more sugar and carbohydrate one eats the more allergy thrives, so remember to restrict or preferably remove from your diet all sugars and refined carbohydrates and concentrate more on raw foods, fruits, limited amounts of dairy produce and large quantities of pure bottled spring water to flush the system out.

When one goes on a fast all allergy disappears, so that is surely proof that allergy comes from within, not without. Reflexology helps enormously with allergic conditions as it encourages the bodily functions to normalize and creates a great feeling of relaxation.

I once treated a patient for his allergic hay fever which was so severe and disabling that life throughout May, June and July was not worth living. His hay fever usually also created an asthmatic condition as the weeks proceeded. Reflexology treatments helped, but I did encourage him to spend a holiday at a certain health farm. He arrived at this beautiful centre and was quite dismayed to find the masses of roses all out in full flower. The perfume was intense, and so was the pollen. Within hours an asthma attack occured and the local doctor was summoned. He treated the condition with a steroid injection. The doctor at the health farm suggested that he have a complete bowel wash-out to rid the body of all its impurities, and he then fasted for a week on nothing but grapes and spring water. At the end of that week there was no sign at all of any allergy and the patient felt really well. At the request of the doctor and much to his horror he was taken back to that dreaded mass of roses, the doctor asked him to inhale the perfume, which he did, and there was no reaction at all – proof indeed that once the body is detoxified, allergy and disease fail to manifest.

Conservative estimates indicate that 75 per cent of illnesses are psychosomatic. Psychsomatic does not mean that the illness does not exist in reality. It simply means that illness is caused by the action of the mind (psyche) on the body (soma). Nevertheless, dietary care has a dynamic effect on health. We are exactly what we eat. After all, the body was formed from and is fuelled by food but whatever condition you are tackling remember that emotions form a great part in causing disease and a positive mental attitude has a great effect on the healing processes.

# 4  Energies

When one considers the word 'energies' I am sure it conjures up many strange and mystical connotations. You may think that energy relates to an extremely active person, or some sinister picture may be formed of witchcraft or spiritualism. Just as we have atmospheric energies in our universe, such as television, radio, radar, electricity and so on, man also has a powerful life force or energy radiating throughout his entire being. This energy is the greatest controlling influence of our life. It can be used to destroy or create.

How can something that is invisible control our lives, you may ask. Well, what about the power of the mind? It you delved surgically into the brain, you cannot cut out mind and lay it upon a plate. Yet our thinking power, which is our mind, is the governor of our life. We talk of a soulful person (positive) or a soulless individual (negative). There is an immutable law which says, 'As within, so without; cause and effect'. In other words, the thought forces, the various mental states and the emotions all have, in the long term, their effects upon the physical body.

You may doubt a great deal what is said today with regard to the effects of the mind upon the body. Someone brings you sudden news, you grow pale, you tremble, or perhaps you fall into a faint. It is, however, through the channel of your mind that the news is imparted to you.

A friend says something to you, perhaps at table, something that seems very unkind. You are hurt by this remark. You have been enjoying your meal, but from that moment your appetite is gone. What was said entered into and affected you through the channel of your mind.

Again, a sudden emergency arises. You stand, unable to move, weak with fear. What causes the trembling? And yet you believe that the mind has but little influence upon the body. You are for a few moments dominated by anger. For hours afterwards you complain of a violent headache. Fear and worry have the effect of closing up the channels of the body so that the life forces flow in a slow and sluggish manner. Hope and tranquillity open the channels of the body so that the life forces go bounding through it in such a way that disease can rarely get a foothold.

I always remember a patient of mine who came with a sudden onset of a very disabling form of arthritis that had reduced her from a fit, active woman to one who spent much of her day in an armchair, unable to walk because of pain. It has been proven that most forms of arthritis are influenced by suppression of anger throughout life – some sudden shock, suppressed grief or the inability to accept or tolerate a certain situation that has cropped up in one's life. I gave this lady her first treatment of reflexology and tried to delve into her past. With great difficulty I eventually got her to talk about a certain very painful situation that had occurred just nine months before, three months prior to the onset of her illness. Her only and much-loved son had fallen in love with a young lady whom she disliked intensely. She felt sure her son had made a wrong choice and could not bear the thought of his marrying this girl and leaving her alone. Her mind had become so poisoned about their relationship, she was so beset with jealousy and, in a way, grief, that she turned her body into the acid condition that stimulated the onset of the arthritis.

I explained as best I could the effect of the mind upon her body, asked if she realized that apart from the bad relationship she now had with both her son and daughter-in-law, she in fact, was the one who sat alone in pain, not them. I also told her that no matter how many reflexology treatments she had from me, I could only relieve her pain: the cause of the problem was in her own hands and that it was up to her to change these terrible, destructive, negative thoughts, and try to make peace with her son and his new wife.

I treated her for three months and emotionally supported her through her mental and physical healing crises. She did come to terms with the situation and eventually became quite friendly with her daughter-in-law. Within that year she was back to her fit active self with no trace of arthritis. She swore it was the reflexology that helped, but the 'cure' was her change of attitude, the peace that returned to her soul.

I always remember the statement made by a famous scientist, Michael Faraday, who invented the first dynamo. 'It is known that all matter is composed of atoms vibrating at different rates to form different densities, but what we should also know is that all matter of any substance owes whatever it may possess to the types of electrical charge or vibration given off by that substance.'

Any good book on physics will tell you that energy cannot be destroyed but that it can travel. It cannot be seen since it is invisible, but it can leave the body and as it leaves we become weaker and weaker. If you have ever talked with anyone who has had a heart attack he will tell you that his energy seemed to drain away and he was lifeless. The body is based on an electrical circuit, and like normal electrical circuits it has its negative and positive poles. The heart represents the negative, the brain the positive, but there should be balance between the heart and the brain.

Reflexology is a method of contacting the electrical centres in the body. Balance and order must be created before health becomes established. Reflexology has been used for centuries to create a smooth flow of vibratory energy through the body by contacting various points in the feet which relate to various organs, glands and cells.

We all have a dynamic power of healing; we all have this 'life force' or 'energy' which radiates through our bodies and can be channelled to heal. I would like you to concentrate for a few moments on your hands, since they convey important sensory information. Rub your hands together; feel the sensation like an electric charge. Now close your eyes and try an energy-sensing exercise with your hands. Rub them together gently and when you feel a warmth stop rubbing. Now slowly move your hands a few inches apart. If you feel a warmth or energy flow develop between them, move them even further apart and then closer together again. Observe any change in sensation as your hands move apart and then back together again. It may take time for the energy flow to develop or for you to recognize what is already there. You may experience a force field as your hands approach each other. As you become aware of the 'power in your hands' you will be able to feel this energy flow when your hands are far apart. You may also experience a 'tingling sensation' in your palms or fingertips, a feeling as if your hands were coming alive.

We sometimes hear a person in poor health say to another, 'I always feel better when you come.' The power of suggestion so far as the human mind is concerned is a most wonderful and interesting field of study.

It has been proved from laboratory experiments that the entire human structure can be completely changed, made over, within a period of less than one year, and that in some portions the cells are entirely replaced within a period of a very few weeks.

We must all remember that health is contagious as well as disease, and it is up to each one of us to take responsibility for our own health and realize that we can either infuse ourselves with a positive life force energy or 'join forces with the devil'.

I expect most of you will have experienced death at some time in your life. You may have lost a much-loved relative, or even an animal, and will have observed that at death all that is left is a worn-out shell. The very special something that you will remember about that person has left the body. This is your life force or the dynamic energy that can be channelled into the power of healing.

Perhaps we can all now begin to understand the principles of the laying on of hands and how in all the portrayals of Christ and his disciples in works of art, great attention is paid to the hands. Hands are held high above the heads of sinners, hands are placed on the bodies of the sick. In all these instances the hands are channelling this loving, vital energy into those depleted of it. Hands were really meant for healing; healing was meant to be gentle, simple and passive in all its forms. We, as reflexologists can give all these things through our treatment of those very vital sensitive reflex points in the feet which manifest through the vital pathways of the body.

Many a writer, composer or artist will tell you that there have been occasions during his life when all attempts to write, compose or paint were impossible and that he felt dead inside. These occasions were when he was 'out of tune' with life and had become disconnected from life's energy forces.

My final example or explanation of this divine energy force that radiates throughout each and every one of us is the so-called 'body chemistry' that is emitted and attracts others. This very powerful attraction between two people causes them to feel 'at one'. We refer to this interaction as 'falling in love.' When one feels at peace and a oneness with another it is actually this weaving together of the powerful energy of life.

The wonderful thing about learning to practise reflexology is that it is available for everybody. You don't have to have a medical qualification or even be involved in the medical profession at all. The qualifications needed are a warm, compassionate nature, a true empathy towards the sick and that very special asset, the motivation to learn slowly the principles of reflexology, the true understanding of holistic healing and a good background knowledge of the history of natural medicine. You will develop the power in your hands as you begin to study through the courses the practical application of working upon the feet, with a very fine, slow, deep pressure therapy which you will apply with your thumb and index finger. This technique you have to learn at a training course. It is impossible to learn with just the aid of a book.

Some of us have more potential to develop the skills of reflexology than others. The same applies to any other medical science, but I have found in my vast experience that in general those sensitive, intuitive types of people who are frequently found to be very creative either in the field of music, art, literature, sculpture and – strange as it may seem – those who have 'green fingers' become very sensitive in their skills as a reflexologist and many other natural therapies.

# 5 Stress

Reflexology has a dynamic effect on the body in its ability to relieve stress and tension. It also improves nerve and blood supply and restores the body back into a state of normality and balance, so whether it is a build-up of emotional tensions which have put the body into a state of disharmony or a situation of physical stress you can be sure of some very quick, effective results, even after only two or three treatment sessions.

Stress plays a very destructive part in breaking down the defence mechanisms in the body. Most of us evaluate stress in relation to a business executive or a 'high flyer'. I am therefore going to devote this chapter to explaining the real meaning of stress and its effect upon the body.

To start with, stress does not have to be 'all bad': there are situations in life when it is essential for our bodies to cope with the demands sometimes made on them. In its primitive form stress is the 'fight or flight' reaction, and instantly the body prepares to do battle or run, hormones are released into the bloodstream, which encourage all the systems in the body to work to their ultimate. It also releases fuel in the form of glucose or stored blood sugar. More blood is sent to the muscles, the air passages become relaxed and a sense of stimulation is produced.

When one is in an acutely stressful situation it is common to experience frequent bowel actions and an increase in the urine output. This reaction is again very primitive in its origin, as, in order for man to flee or fight, it was necessary for the body to be as weightless as possible.

There are everyday tensions that we have to learn to cope with, commuting on a crowded train, contending with a snarling boss, wondering how to keep on the right side of a fussy husband or a bossy wife. Such stresses are minor only in that they do not immediately transform our lives, as would the death of, say, a spouse or a gaol sentence. However, the naggingly persistent daily stresses affect the body and make it more vulnerable to disease than do acute traumatic situations.

Stress is not all black or distressing; in fact, some forms of stress are immensely stimulating. An athlete or mountaineer subjects himself to stress; stress is a part of achieving, of experiencing life's ultimate sensations. A pianist accompanying, say, the London Philharmonic Orchestra, can be so involved in the emotional euphoria of his interpretation of the music that sweat pours off his face, adrenalin pumps around his circulation, his heart pounds. This is the human machine seen at its very best, at the peak of creative coordination. This is the kind of intense short-term stress which evolution has equipped us to cope with.

Many psychologists agree that people with a past history of traumatic stress experiences are likely to react adversely to similar future stress encounters. A latent traumatic experience may go undetected for many years until a new crisis revives the feelings and ideas related to the original trauma. These subjects are likely to demonstrate far more anxiety, greater physiological stress reactivity and poorer intellectual functioning under new yet similar traumatic circumstances than people with no such experience.

Reassuringly, however, even during the last few years there has been a major change of ideas within psychology and psychiatry about concepts such as 'normality' and 'insanity'. Gone are the days when those exhibiting bizarre behavioural episodes were certified 'insane' and spent the rest of their lives in asylums.

A team of monks in Canada headed by a psychologist researched into patients suffering from schizophrenia, and found in the main that these patients were extremely psychic and were in fact 'tuned in' to a higher spiritual level, which explained the voices which they heard and which ultimately governed their behaviour. It was concluded that the higher spiritual power was of very 'negative' origin.

Psychological discomfort can arise in many stressful ways. You may feel guilt from an illicit love affair, tension in times of crisis, hopelessness in times of loss, or anxiety caused by work or monetary situations. Some people seek the comfort of religion, though religion is no longer the powerful solace it once was. Most would far rather turn to medically prescribed drugs which make them feel 'numbed', and the suffering is then not so acute. Nobody is prepare to relinquish the cause of stress or wait for nature to take its course.

Sadly, the taking of tranquillizers or sleeping pills has become a dominant part of life for an increasing number of people. Such people use drugs to stay awake, go to sleep, or as a general prop for everyday living. Problems are no longer confronted and coped with but are set aside and left unresolved. Even non-addicted people who lean on temporary psychological props during an emotional upheaval often find it difficult to break the pill-popping habit.

Living in our commercial, fast-paced society is stress-provoking. Traffic, television, noise, job pressures to get ahead, family problems and so on set up states of alarm in our bodies with great frequency. The body responds automatically to stress situations. Physiological changes take place that prepare the body for fight or flight. Without conscious effort we become ready for action, geared to do something about the stressful situation that the body perceives. The great frustration is that usually no action is taken. One cannot strike the boss, and it is not usual to run away from one's family. Modern society evokes alarms in us that are inappropriate because action responses can seldom be made that are socially unacceptable.

In the Western world, rapidly increasing numbers of people are afflicted with high blood pressure, heart attacks and strokes. Mounting stress and the many causes of fatigue are certainly some of the important causes of these illnesses. Frank Ward O'Malley noted that 'Life is just one damned thing after another.' Changes in our society come about quite slowly, but there are changes we can bring about in ourselves which can be done fairly quickly.

When an individual learns to relax habitually, he has less need for fight or flight reactions. He may well be a less hostile person and he often feels better about himself as a person. He is often better able to confront problems in his life because he has a mechanism of handling uptight feelings. He is often able to solve problems that eluded him previously. That is why meditation is becoming a popular method of bringing about a relaxed state in mind and body.

The yogis used to practise transcendental meditation by concentrating upon the flame of a candle. Coal and log fires are unfortunately not so popular, but if you do have one, concentrate your attention on watching the flickering flames and you should, within about fifteen minutes, experience an acute drowsy sensation, begin yawning and fall asleep very easily. Yawning has the effect of relaxing tension in any case, and if we refer to the zones in our reflexology learning (see page 37), we can perhaps understand that as we yawn we stimulate through our jaw, head and face the ten zones in our system. An acutely anxious person frequently yawns, which is nature's way of helping him reduce his stress level.

People who meditate can withstand more life changes with the development of less illness. Furthermore, experienced meditators have the least illness of all. Something about meditation helps the individual to cope with life's problems. There is an extra gain obtained from fatigue-relieving meditation. Because the mind is trained to focus on one thing to the exclusion of all else, the capacity to pay attention improves. This focusing of attention occurs with relaxation.

Long-term symptoms of constant fatigue are symptoms of an anxiety state, or those of depression. The nervous system becomes so drained and depleted that the only physical reaction is fatigue, which will make the person choose to opt out of everything. Depression can be a disturbance caused by situations of suppressed rage as a child. Anger is a normal reaction, so are tears, but we as a nation are generally very repressed. The best way of coping with anger is to throw, if you have them, a pile of old cracked plates against a wall; the noise is very mentally satisfying. Or punch the living daylights out of a bale of hay, which you can keep in the seclusion and privacy of your garage. Otherwise, a heavy game of squash, tennis or some excess physical activity are all excellent ways of coping with stress. What you should learn not to do is to work out your anger by violence on another person. All too frequently this happens in society today.

Unrelentingly unchanging jobs, dissatisfaction with life, lack of challenge, and dull, unimaginative associates may contribute to boredom which brings on fatigue. To wake tired after a full night's sleep is a common symptom in the depressed individual. Low blood sugar may contribute to the depressive's symptoms and should be checked out first by the usual blood investigations. The depressed individual may have, in addition to fatigue, feelings of hopelessness, guilt, poor self-esteem and somatic symptoms such as sleep disturbance, constipation and loss of appetite. Suicide is a distinct possibility in any patient who has a serious clinical depression.

The need to perform at a level above one's capacity may easily produce fatigue. Often, too, in this situation some physical illness will occur and serve as a justifiable reason for escaping from such pressure. Equally, performing much below one's capabilities may be equally productive of fatigue. In this case, frustration, disappointment and bottled-up anger may underlie the fatigue.

In successful achievement of a task there may be greater use of mind and body than in failure. Success on the job may leave one tired yet exhilarated, whereas failure may put one to bed for a week. There is a distinct mental aspect to the tolerance of fatigue. When one is winning a tennis match a player is likely to be able to play on through his fatigue; when losing he is apt to default from fatigue. When the distance runner grows tired at the end of a race he may yet find that extra energy for a final spurt of speed. His ability to command this extra energy is dependent, in part, on his mental attitude.

Many people today suffer from anxiety neurosis. Medical examination reveals no organic cause and the individual is declared healthy. These poor sufferers have an overwhelming feeling of anxiety and their minds are continually churning. They perspire, suffer from heart palpitations, muscular aches and pains and frightening attacks of breathlessness. In acute cases they may begin hyperventilating, which leads to an episode of unconsciousness. Psychiatrists often refer to this as an 'hysterical overlay', it is in a way nature offering her own anaesthetic, to enable the patient to break away from the intolerable circumstance in which he finds himself. In these situations the patient almost longs for something to be found medically to explain his symptoms, and so the declaration that nothing abnormal has been found gives rise to even more panic.

You may, if you are a therapist, be approached by people who suffer from insomnia, and you may, if you are a sufferer, seek out a reflexologist to help you with this unpleasant state. A few special causes of insomnia exist, but in 95 per cent of cases, sleep difficulties can be traced to underlying anxiety or depression. People who are depressed sleep for only a few hours and wake up very early. Many cases of insomnia and consequently depression are now thought to be due to biochemical imbalances, and they may even be partly hereditary.

You will surely meet many people suffering from the conditions and symptoms that I have mentioned in this chapter. Never be afraid to treat any stress situation, as they respond well to regular reflexology treatments.

Reflexology does create a sensation of well-being. This alone can enable those suffering from anxiety states to have some respite from their symptoms. Although we cannot change people's thinking, we can perhaps enable them to approach situations in a different light because of the improvement in their state of tension.

# 6 The history of zone therapy

Dr William Fitzgerald, the founder of Zone Therapy, was born in Middletown, Connecticut, USA, in 1872. He graduated in medicine from the University of Vermont in 1895 and then spent some years in hospitals in Vienna, Paris and London. He later practised in the Hospital for Diseases of the Ear, Nose and Throat in Hartford, Connecticut, then transferred his practice and teaching to New York and died in Stamford in 1942.

Developing the work of Dr H. Bressler, Dr Fitzgerald went to Vienna in the early part of this century to consider the possibility of treating organs through pressure points. In his book *Zone Therapy* he makes some interesting remarks about its history: 'A form of treatment by means of pressure point was known in India and China some 5,000 years ago. This knowledge appears however to have been lost or forgotten, perhaps it was set aside in favor of acupuncture, which emerged as the stronger growth from the same root.'

In central European countries similar methods had been described in 1582 by the physicians Adamus and A'Tatis. The great Florentine sculptor Benvenuto Cellini (1500–1571) used strong pressure on his fingers and toes to relieve pain anywhere in his body, with remarkable success.

The twentieth American President, James A. Garfield (1831–1881) was able to alleviate the pains he had following an assassination attempt by applying pressure to various points in his feet. No other pain-killing medicines gave him relief. The relationship between reflex points and the internal organs of the body was known by various North American Indian tribes and this knowledge was used in the treatment of disease. This knowledge has been preserved over many centuries and is still used in India for the relief of pain.

We all use a form of pressure therapy in an attempt to relieve pain, and I am sure we are aware of exactly what we do when we clench our teeth when in extreme pain, when we apply pressure to our temples when suffering a severe headache. When we bang our elbow against a door or piece of furniture, we instinctively apply pressure to the injured part with the corresponding hand. We are using pressure to relieve pain. When a child falls and hurts his knee, we pick him up and rub it better.

In 1916 Dr Edwin Bowers first publicly described the treatment nurtured by Dr Fitzgerald, and called it 'zone therapy'. One year later their combined work appeared in the book *Zone Therapy*, which contained medical recommendations for doctors, dentists, gynaecologists, ENT specialists and chiropractors. According to Dr George Starr White in 1925, the fact that zone therapy was probably more widely known throughout the United States than elsewhere was evidence indeed that the foundation of the work was solid.

Dr Fitzgerald gave courses of instruction and gathered about him a circle of practitioners. Diagrams of the zones of the feet and the corresponding division of the ten zones of the body appeared in the first edition of his book.

Dr Fitzgerald also found that if pressure upon the fingers was applied, it could create a local anaesthetic effect to the hand, arm, and shoulder right up into the jaw, face, ear and nose. He applied the pressure by using tight bands of elastic on the middle section of each finger, or small clamps which he placed upon the tips. By this intervention he was able to carry out minor surgical operations just using this pressure technique. This finding has similarities to the operations that have been undertaken in recent years, whereby the only means of anaesthesia were acupuncture needles which, when placed in prime positions, created a local anaesthetic effect to the organ or part being operated upon.

Acupuncture was first introduced into Western medicine in 1883 when the Dutch physician Ten Thyne wrote a treatise on the subject. In the early nineteenth century Berlioz, physician and father of the composer, published a positive account of the results he had with zone therapy treatment, which at that time was being used by at least some physicians.

In 1898 the English neurologist Henry Head discovered zones on the skin which became hypersensitive to pressure when an organ connected by nerves to this skin region was diseased. These zones were named after him. In more recent years Russian physiologists have carried out extensive studies using encephalography, electrocardiography and X-ray. Studies involving the measurement of the electrical potential of the skin at the classical acupuncture points have verified basic claims for acupuncture and have related its effect to reflex action. The skin might be thought of as a screen on which the inner organs are projected through nerve connections as part of a telephone relay system in which the stimulation of a certain point by pressure – or as in acupuncture, by a prick – spreads through the reflex action to the nerve-connected inner organ. There are about 690 acupuncture points on the skin, clustering along fourteen major lines of the body on to the feet in the right location.

Three lateral zones are commonly used in reflexology, the diaphragm line, waist line and heel line and also ten vertical zones (see Figure 1). The right foot corresponds to the right side of the body and the left foot corresponds to the left. If we can visualize the body being sliced in half, just like cutting through an apple, the centre being the nose, we can perhaps imagine that the reflexes do go directly through the body.

You must have all noticed how animals constantly lick their newborn. The licking is not for reasons of cleanliness alone. The constant licking of the fur of the newborn animal stimulates the nerve impulses through the zones on the surface of the body, which in turn causes a reaction to the organs, encouraging the bodily functions to mature.

A gall bladder fistula was experimentally induced in a horse by a Romanian team of investigators, and when a point said to be related to the gall bladder was pricked there was an increase in the flow of bile. This did not occur when other skin points were pricked.

Professor Bresson, attached to a veterinary medical institute, conducted a five-year study using dogs, cats and horses. Animals that had not responded to the usual treatments responded well to acupuncture. The success of acupuncture on animals, which is still based on working on certain zones or

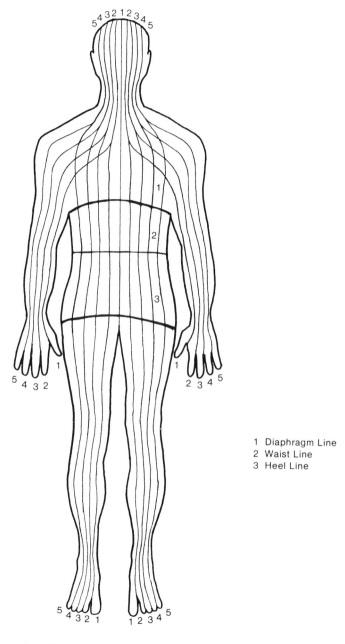

1 Diaphragm Line
2 Waist Line
3 Heel Line

*Figure 1   Body zones*

lines in the body, should dispel any notion that positive results are due to a suggestive influence of treatment.

It was the Chinese who, beginning with an accidental occurrence which has certainly been experienced by people in other parts of the world, discovered that pain disappeared when a point on the skin was pricked. They followed up their observations and developed them into the Chinese art of healing. By the early 1930s the time had come for the further refinement of zone therapy into foot reflexology.

Dr George Shelby Riley's therapy assistant, Eunice Ingham, had been using the zone therapy system in her work but began to feel that the feet should be the specific area for therapy because of their highly sensitive nature. She charted the feet in relation to the zones and their effects on the rest of the anatomy until finally she had evolved on the feet themselves a 'map' of the entire body. She found that instead of applying constant direct pressure she could use an alternating pressure; this seemed to have remarkable effects beyond pain reduction. She was so successful that her reputation soon spread and she became known as the 'foot therapist'.

She wrote her first book in 1938, *Stories the Feet Can Tell*, and is now recognized as the founder of foot reflexology. She retired in 1970. Her niece, Eusebia Messenger, and nephew, Dwight Byers, continued to promote her work.

Zone therapy is therefore the basis of foot reflexology. Reflexology has become a more refined system, but an understanding of the zones is essential in order to understand reflexology.

There are ten equal longitudinal zones running the length of the body from the top of the head to the tips of the toes. The number ten corresponds to the fingers and toes and therefore provides a simple numbering system. Each finger and toe falls into one zone, with the fifth toe occurring in the same zone as the fifth finger.

If you shut your eyes and trace ten zones on your own body it will simplify my explanation. Start with your big toe and trace a line from the toe through the leg, the trunk and chest and right up in line with your nose. now reverse the procedure and start imagining a line running from your thumb to your big toe. Each big toe corresponds to half of the head area. Congestion or tension in any part of a zone will affect the entire zone, running through the whole length of the body. Any organ, gland or function throughout that zone may be out of order. Someone you know may often complain of trouble on his or her right side; the right side of the neck or perhaps the right shoulder is painful. Maybe it is the right hip and knee. Why is it so? The reason is simply, as I have explained, that when one part of a zone is affected it ultimately creates a problem throughout its entire length.

Sensitivity in a specific part of the foot is a signal to the reflexologist that there is congestion or inflammation in that zone. Direct pressure applied through the foot will affect the entire zonal area from foot to head.

I want you to place your naked feet firmly in front of you, observe how perfectly the feet 'mirror' the body. The five toes on the right foot govern the head and shoulder areas on the right, the upper section of the foot from the diaphragm contains reflexes that affect the organs in the upper part of the body, the chest, lung and breast area. The middle section of the foot from the waist line to the diaphragm has reflex points to the liver, kidneys, stomach and pancreas areas. From the waist line to the heel line we find the reflex points to the intestinal areas.

Now separate your feet and turn them outwards. We are basically cutting the body in half. As your spine is in the middle zone of your body, its relative reflex area must be on the inside edge of both feet, and it is (see Figure 2b). Any organ or part that is in the midline or first zone of the body, such as the uterus, will have its reflex point on the inside edge of both feet.

Understandably, and quite reasonably, many people are initially sceptical and even bewildered when we begin to apply this pressure therapy to their feet. They can see no connection between their ailments and the treatment of their feet. Today, however, with an increasing interest in acupuncture and acupressure there is a growing readiness to believe that interrelationships exist between certain points of the body and organs widely removed from such points. Because of the

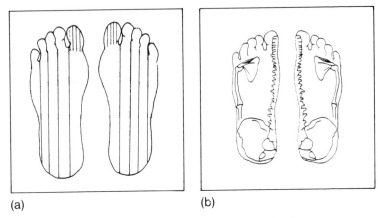

(a)                    (b)

*Figure 2    a) Zones relating to the feet; b) skeletal areas*

acceptance of acupuncture a similar relationship between certain areas of the feet and the body is now at least open to question. The great feeling of well-being and, indeed, the reactions that most people receive after a treatment session have been instrumental in bringing about a change of thinking in a very short space of time.

Reflexology is not the panacea to all health problems of man. No single science has been, or will ever be. I have found in my vast experience over these ten years during which I have been fully involved in the treatment of patients and training of reflexologists, that all the everyday conditions for which one goes to a doctor's surgery can be greatly relieved or removed altogether with frequent treatments of reflexology over a short period of time. Migraine, asthma, bronchitis, digestive problems, kidney and bladder conditions, high blood pressure – all these respond admirably. I would say that top on the list of success is the treatment of all back pain problems, and as back conditions are almost epidemic in proportion, we can be sure of a ready flow of sufferers who will seek out, in desperation, a reflexologist to help them.

I am sure you realize now that reflexology is a logical, safe and very effective science.

# 7 The digestive system

The digestive system consists of the alimentary canal and certain associated organs which are involved in the chewing, swallowing, breakdown and absorption of food as well as the expulsion from the body of what is left after these processes are complete.

In the mouth food is bathed in amylase-rich secretions of the salivary glands and mastication, involving teeth and tongue, breaks it up. With starch digestion already under way the food is transferred to the next part of the alimentary tract by the reflex action of swallowing. The food reaches the oesophagus in about ten seconds and passes into the stomach, which has a reservoir function and can hold some 1,500 ml in the adult. Here it is minutely divided by churning peristaltic contraction waves and also mixed with gastric juice to form a paste called chyme. Gastric juice is rich in hydrochloric acid and the protein-splitting enzyme pepsin. The rate of gastric emptying depends on the degree of distension and the type of food ingested.

A muscular valve, the pyloris, controls the emptying process by opening after every four to five peristaltic waves. In the duodenum the chyme is exposed to the pancreatic juice, which contains further carbohydrate, protein and fat-splitting enzymes. The effect of the latter is helped considerably by the mixture of bile secreted from the liver.

During transit through the small intestine the products of these digestive processes are absorbed both actively and passively, and transported directly to the liver in the portal venous system.

The liver is the largest gland in the body and receives some 1.5 litres of blood per minute. The liver cells have vital functions in storage and recombination of digestive products, the inactivation of hormones, the detoxification of drugs and poisons and the formation and excretion of bile. The 1.5 m of large intestine running from the ileocecal valve to the anus or

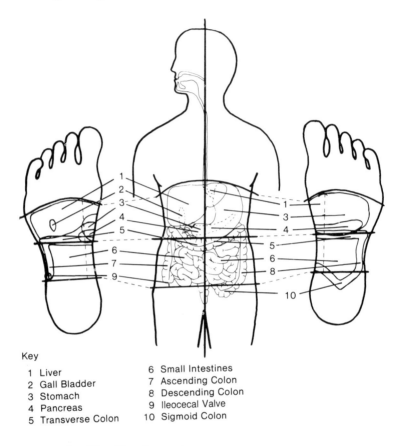

Key

1 Liver
2 Gall Bladder
3 Stomach
4 Pancreas
5 Transverse Colon

6 Small Intestines
7 Ascending Colon
8 Descending Colon
9 Ileocecal Valve
10 Sigmoid Colon

*Figure 3   The digestive system*

rectum completes the 9 m of alimentary tract. Its functions are related mainly to the absorption of water and electrolyte irons. The unabsorbable residue is concentrated in the descending colon as faecal matter, which is discharged through the anal canal by the voluntary act of defecation. Despite wide differences in function, each section of the alimentary canal has the same basic structure, strongly supported by muscle fibres.

Within the mouth we have three main pairs of salivary glands, parotid, sublingual and submandibular.

The stomach is the most dilated part of the digestive tract and lies in the upper left part of the abdomen. It has two curvatures, lesser and greater, two surfaces, anterior and posterior, and two orfices, cardiac and pyloric. The functions of the stomach are to act as a reservoir for food, to prepare it for entry into the intestines by warming, mixing and initiating digestion and to pass it into the duodenum in appropriate amounts. The reservoir function is performed mainly by relaxation of muscular fibres in the body. At the distal end of the stomach the pyloric sphincter is a thickened part of the stomach's inner circular muscle layer.

The liver weighs between 1.2 and 1.8 kg in the adult, lies in the right side of the upper abdomen and has two lobes, the left much smaller than the right. Although firm to the touch, liver tissue is extremely friable because of the organ's great vascularity. At the periphery of each lobule are several portal tracts containing branches of the hepatic artery, portal vein and bile ducts, together with fibrous connective tissue and small lymphatics. The blood supply to the liver is a mixed venous and arterial one. Although only a fifth of the supply is derived from the hepatic artery this source provides half its oxygen requirements. The most common condition which severely affects the liver is cirrhosis associated with poor nutrition and or a high alcohol intake.

The liver produces bile, which is stored and secreted by the gall bladder. The bile is produced from the breakdown of haemoglobin, bile acids and salts and mucin. Bile salts emulsify fat and therefore assist in the absorption of dietary fat and fat-soluble vitamins. Bile also constitutes an important exit pathway for certain drugs and poisons. Some 500 ml of bile is excreted every day.

The pancreas is about 15 cm long and lies across the posterior wall of the abdomen between the curve of the duodenum and splenic hilum. It has an alkaline exocrine secretion, pancreatic juice which is discharged into the duodenum via the pancreatic duct. Scattered throughout the serous exocrine glandular tissue are small islets of specialized endocrine cells (Islets of Langerhans) which, although occupying only about 1 per cent of the pancreatic mass, are vital to carbohydrate metabolism. The alpha cells produce glucagon; the beta cells secrete insulin.

Failure of insulin production leads to the clinical condition of diabetes mellitus.

The intestine can simply be summarized as a tube of great flexible structure. It is divided conveniently into two parts: the small intestine, which extends from the pyloric valve to the ileocecal junction; and the large intestine, which runs from the ileocecal junction to the anus. The small intestine, some 6–7 m long, begins with 25 cm of duodenum. This curves around the head of the pancreas. The duodenal mucous membrane is thrown into crescent-shaped folds which project into the bowel to retard the progress of chyme as well as offering an increased area for absorption. The duodenum runs on into the jejunum and ileum.

The large intestine is much larger than the small intestine in width, but much shorter in length – some 1.5 m. Unlike the small intestine it is relatively fixed in position. Commencing from the caecum the ascending colon becomes transverse at the right hepatic flexure, then turns downwards into the descending colon at the left splenic flexure. Passing into the lesser pelvis this forms a curving loop, the sigmoid colon, before dilating into the rectum and anal canal. Some 3 cm from the ileocecal valve lies the base of the appendix. Of variable length and position, this blind-ended narrow tube is rich in lymphoid tissue. Although frequently the site of obstruction and inflammation the diagnosis of acute appendicitis can be very difficult to make because of these variations.

An enormous number of deaths occur each year as the result of diseases affecting the digestive system. Reflexology offers some excellent results in helping the healing process in the body.

You will see that I have identified in Figure 3 the reflex areas in the feet that relate to the parts of the body that we have mentioned. There will be extreme sensitivity in all the areas relating to the digestive system if there is a disorder or disfunction in any part of the digestive system.

I have treated patients suffering from ulceration of the duodenum and stomach, and within a very short period of time they have been freed from a lot of pain and felt generally much improved in their health. There has been great success also in those suffering from the distressing condition of colitis, and those sufferers from the common condition, constipation, will have great relief from this unpleasant state which causes much disease throughout the body. I always remember an old doctor saying to me, 'You never find flies around a clean dustbin.' If the bowel contains a mass of digested food that is not eliminated regularly, it must be obvious that a very toxic state can occur in the body.

I remember a young schoolteacher who came to me with a history of diverticulitis for many years. She was constantly on medication to relieve her symptoms. When she came to my clinic she was in a very weak state having had almost constant diarrhoea for two weeks which did not seem to be controlled by the medication which was prescribed for her. Upon commencing work on her feet I was amazed at the sensitivity that was apparent in the transverse and descending colon on the left foot. Even the lightest pressure on these very sensitive reflex points caused tears to come into her eyes. The sensitivity continued right down into the sigmoid part of the colon.

It was obvious to me that this acute sensitivity must indicate that the colon was in a very bad condition. I felt that here was a serious condition that was beyond the help of reflexology. I suggested to the teacher that she see her doctor in the morning and ask for a letter to see a specialist. Within a month I had a telephone call from her mother who said that they had taken my advice and had seen a specialist. After extensive investigations it was found that surgery was necessary. The entire descending and sigmoid colon was severely ulcerated, and had surgery not been carried out immediately the patient would have suffered from peritonitis, as the ulcers were, in places, actually discharging into the pelvic cavity. So here was a case where I could offer no help, but the feet did tell a story and revealed so accurately the areas that were in trouble. The teacher was very grateful for my advice and was amazed at the accuracy that could be detected from the feet.

I always say to my students, 'You will never be able to help "the world" but a very great proportion of it.'

# 8 The reproductive system

The reproductive system consists of the uterus, ovaries and fallopian tubes in the female and the testicles, vas deferens and prostate gland in the male. Sex hormones are released by the pituitary gland, so it is essential to work out thoroughly the glandular system when treating cases of infertility, menstrual disorders and menopausal problems.

The time of prenatal development is the period of growth about which we know least. Our ignorance begins at the beginning, with fertilization. We do not know what forces are responsible for selecting out of millions of sperm the one which fertilizes the ovum. After fertilization in one of the tubes leading from the ovaries to the uterus, the fertilized egg spends several days in the tube before implanting itself in the wall of the uterus. During this time the cells divide steadily. About 30 hours after fertilization the ovum divides into two cells, a second division occurs some 20 hours later giving four cells and by the time of implantation there are already about 150 cells.

When the foetus is only six weeks old and 3 cm long it is recognizably human and has a nervous system which shows the beginning of reflex responses to tactile stimuli, a beating heart, arms and legs. Other organs such as the intestines, liver and kidneys are also taking shape, as are the eyes, ears, mouth and nostrils. Never again does the human body grow at such a speed as during this early dynamic phase.

The uterus, a muscular organ, is situated in the mid-pelvic area between the bladder and the rectum. A full bladder will tilt it backward and a distended rectum will tilt it forward. You will see therefore how many bladder and colon problems can have an effect on the uterus, and frequently by helping a chronic case of constipation, uterine problems will disappear.

During the first 24 weeks in the uterus the accumulation of protein accounts for most of the rise in foetal weight. Thereafter the foetus stores considerable amounts of energy in the form of

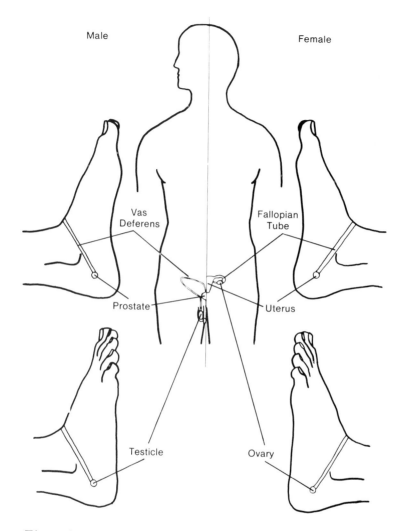

*Figure 4    The reproductive system*

fat in preparation for the post birth period. Analysing 36 foetuses at this age Drs D. A. T. Southgate and E. Hay found that fat increased from 30 g to 430 g between about 30 and 40 weeks.

It seems that the pace of foetal growth slows down from about 34 weeks onwards as available space in the uterus fills up. This braking mechanism ensures that a large baby in the uterus of a small mother can be delivered successfully.

The gonadotrophins released by the pituitary are the same in both sexes and they act in essentially the same way. One of them, follicle stimulating hormone, or FSH, controls the formation of ova or eggs by the ovary and sperm by the testes so it is principally responsible for the propagation of the species. The other is luteinizing hormone, LH, which stimulates the production of sex hormones. There are three groups of sex hormones, androgens, oestrogens and progestogens. All three exist in both sexes, their differing proportions determining gender. Male characteristics, such as a deep voice, facial hair and muscular physique, develop if androgens predominate. The oestrogens on the other hand promote female characteristics such as breast development. The sex hormones also trigger the onset of puberty when sexual identity is given sharper definition.

Theories abound as to the cause of premenstrual tension (PMT) but no one theory seems to apply to all cases of this distressing aspect of the menstrual cycle. It might be that thoughts and fears about PMT compound any problems which occur. Thoughts can and do trigger the secretion of hormones just as they can and do suppress secretion. Tests have shown that women who score high on 'neuroticism tests' tend to suffer more menstrual distress than women who score low. Therefore generally if women expect to suffer from PMT they are more likely to do so. Investigation supports this conclusion. Catholic, Protestant and Jewish women have the same hormonal mechanisms but research has revealed marked differences in their psychological response to menstruation.

Reflexology can help immensely with PMT. I think the greatest benefit results from the degree of relaxation achieved from reflexology treatments and I have had some excellent results with a large number of patients.

One of the best ways of relieving painful menstruation is to swim. Swimming is the only exercise that gives total movement to the whole of the pelvic cavity, and should be used as a regular sport by those suffering from this monthly discomfort.

Combined with reflexology treatment a great all-round improvement can be achieved.

The onset of the menopause can either be extremely trying or symptom free. The most unpleasant symptoms are hot flushes, dizziness, aches and pains in joints and varying mood changes. Reflexology can come to the rescue and greatly help these symptoms.

# 9   The respiratory system

Breathing is regulated by nerve cells in the base of the brain. The trachea (windpipe) descends vertically for about 12 cm and then divides into airways called the bronchi. These then subdivide into much smaller airways, the bronchioles, which carry air into the alveolar ducts of the lungs. Together both lungs weigh about 1.1 kg. The top of each lung reaches to just above the collar bone, and the bases of the lungs end at the last rib.

Bronchitis and emphysema are the most common lung diseases. Acute bronchitis usually lasts only a few days, whereas sufferers from chronic bronchitis eventually experience a great disability from this killing disease. Approximately 20,000 people a year die from chronic bronchitis, and cigarette smoke is the most common bronchial irritant and the major cause of this disease. Those with severe bronchitis may be unable to walk at all. Emphysema (derived from the Greek word meaning 'to puff up') is usually associated with a long history of bronchitis. Because it strikes at the air sacs, causing them to over-inflate and eventually rupture, lung efficiency diminishes. We also know that lung cancer is a most fatal condition of the lung, and 95 per cent of the victims of lung cancer are smokers.

Asthma, an allergic condition which affects the bronchial tubes and lungs, is both a distressing and exhausting condition. It frequently affects the very young and very old.

Reflexology can relieve all problems affecting the respiratory system, and gives quite dramatic results in the treatment of children who seem to respond very quickly after long-term treatments. I am particularly interested in treating children suffering with asthma and bronchitis as I have a son who was almost an invalid as the result of years of asthma and bronchitis and who recovered remarkably through reflexology treatments.

It has been discovered in naturopathic approaches to healing that asthma and all the related 'allergic illness' have their foundations in the digestive system. Allergy has increased

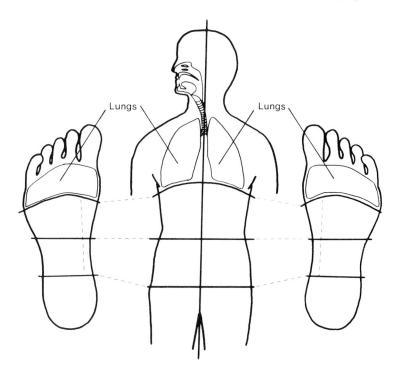

*Figure 5    The respiratory system*

tremendously over the last 25 years and this is due, in the main, to the change in infant feeding procedures. Some infants, we know, have a more delicate digestive system than others, and their stomachs cannot accept wheat and rye products, high-protein cereals and cow's milk. When these infants are fed from an early age on these foods, their digestive systems are not mature enough to cope and therefore set up a resistance or allergy (usually to cow's milk and wheat products). It is quite common for these babies to start on the downward track by having inner ear infections or a constantly runny nose, which of course will be treated by antibiotics. Unfortunately, antibiotics have a directly adverse effect on the intestinal area and so a vicious circle begins: the more infection, the more antibiotics; the more antibiotics, the more 'gumming up' there will be of the intestines. The progression from the runny nose stage is usually

51

to an irritating, wheezing cough which later will be classified as asthma.

The human infant was meant to survive on breast milk and nothing else until it had biting teeth, which usually arrive at the end of the first year, by which time its digestive system has matured sufficiently to start receiving other foods. If any readers of this book have a child in the family suffering from these symptoms, immediately remove the baby from cow's milk and replace with goat's milk, stop all cereal foods and replace with sieved vegetables or fruits, and give no foods or synthetic coloured drinks that contain dyes or additives. Diluted apple or grape juice may be used. Reflexology can give immense relief, and great attention must be paid to working out all the digestive areas, but unless a change in diet is made, no long-term benefit will be obtained.

We can work over the feet of a small baby by just using light pressure over the entire foot. It will of course be impossible to isolate any particular area, but still benefit can be obtained.

In treatment of older children, as long as assistance from the parents in changing the dietary patterns is dealt with and frequent treatments of reflexology are given, there is no reason why the asthma should not be completely removed. Outbreaks of infantile eczema are a warning sign and indicate an irritation within, and should certainly never be treated with cortisone creams and the like which only suppress and drive the inflammation back into the body. Again, however, great attention must be paid to the diet and the same principles followed for those suffering from asthma.

Unfortunately, it is not unusual to find that the asthmatic child lives on a very poor diet and is often, in a way, compensated for his inability to join in sports and for the disabling asthma attacks by being given packets of crisps, cola drinks, bars of chocolate, lollipops and bags of sweets etc. which are unhelpful for his condition. All synthetic sugars and dairy produce – and that includes chocolate – create a mucous condition in the body, and asthmatics already have an abundance of that stored away in their systems.

When treating any case of asthma or bronchitis remember

that the digestive system is the area from which the problem arises, so that is the one to concentrate upon. Work out the kidney and adrenal gland area, then the chest and lung reflex points, which are certainly secondary areas. I have never treated a case of asthma, bronchitis or any other associated condition without finding extreme sensitivity in the intestinal area.

I always remember visiting a daughter of a friend of mine whose child was a chronic asthmatic. Sally was eleven and had been in and out of hospital since the age of three. Her mother was totally sceptical about any form of alternative medicine. When I visited the child she was lying back on her pillows with a face drained of all colour, attached to a steroid drip to control the very severe attack she had just had. There on her locker stood a large bottle of orange squash, a box of dairy milk chocolates and a packet of crisps. I did, eventually, after a lot of hard work, manage to re-educate my friend into the principles and concepts of natural medicine, and explained just how damaging were the junk foods which her sick daughter was eating. She did follow my advice, read some good instructional books and allowed me to treat Sally. It took a lot of hard work and re-education to both parents and the child, but it was successful and one year later Sally was a new child whose asthma attacks became less and less in frequency and were certainly very mild when they did arise. She is now a very attractive teenager who is completely fit and healthy and enjoying a full life. The whole family is fitter also and her parents are true converts to the benefits of reflexology.

# 10   The urinary system

The urinary system contains two kidneys, two ureters (which carry urine from each of the kidneys to the bladder) and the urethra (which is the urinary exit from the bladder). All life is aquatic, and human life is no exception. Although we do not live in water, the cells of our body do. Water accounts for more than half of our body weight. The kidneys maintain the composition and volume of body fluids within very narrow limits. As a result of evolution the urinary and genital tracts have become completely differentiated except for the male urethra, which is the final pathway for both urine and spermatozoa.

The basic unit of the kidney is the nephron. There are some two million nephrons in the paired kidneys, which, with the ureters, bladder and urethra, constitute the urinary system. Homeostasis, the preservation of the body's internal environment in a physiological state of equilibrium, is largely the result of the kidneys' actions. Regulation of the water and electrolyte content, maintenance of the normal acid base equilibrium, elimination of metabolic waste products and retention of vital substances are all features displayed by healthy kidneys. To achieve this remarkable range of functions the kidneys are highly vascular organs, receiving one-quarter of the cardiac output – approximately 1.3 litres per minute. The daily flow of blood through the kidneys is about 1,933 litres, but only about one-thousandth of this is converted into urine; the remainder goes back into the circulation., The two bean-shaped kidneys weigh about 140 g and are buried in fat. They lie close to the spine at the back of the abdomen in front of the twelfth pair of ribs. Each kidney is composed of a million or so nephrons or filters which, if unwound and placed end to end, would stretch for more than 80 kilometres. The filtrate, the basis of urine, passes into the tubules of the nephrons where most of its water and salt content is reabsorbed into the circulation. Of the 170 or so litres of water which filter through

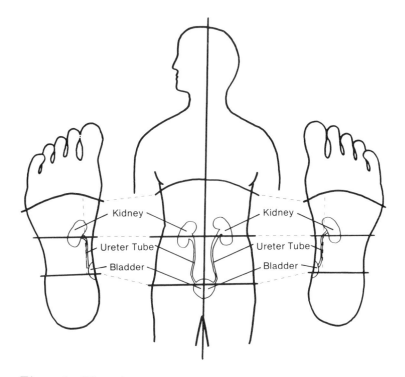

*Figure 6   The urinary system*

the kidneys each day, only about 1½ litres on average are excreted in the urine. If there is too much fluid in the body, the kidneys excrete more; if there is too little, they will excrete less.

The kidneys play an active part in the production of at least three different hormones. For many years it has been known that renin, a hormone involved in the control of blood pressure, is produced by the kidneys, and vitamin D is activated within the kidneys.

The bladder rests in the pelvis, partly protected in the front by the pubic bones. When full it projects up into the abdomen. Urination is controlled by two sphincters, one situated at the exit from the bladder and the other at the exit from the urethra.

Many people, women in particular, suffer from disorders in

the urinary system. In females cystitis, an inflammatory condition of the bladder, is both a painful and lowering condition. The cause can often be a weakness in the vaginal wall due to childbirth or a tendency to infection in the urethra which becomes chronic. These infections can spread and cause infection to the ureter tubes, and eventually the kidneys, which can be very serious indeed. Much can be done to help this condition with reflexology treatments by thoroughly working out the bladder, ureter and kidney areas. Also, attention to the base of the spine and pelvic areas can bring about quite remarkable results. I have treated many cystitis sufferers over the years who all found that reflexology was the only treatment that really gave them any long-term relief. Reflexology can be of great help also in the treatment of an enlarged or inflamed prostate gland in the male.

Remember, when treating patients suffering with high blood pressure, to work out the kidney areas. The kidneys will always be under extreme stress due to the increase of pressure through the arteries in those hypertensive patients.

It is very usual to find sensitivity in patients when one works through the urinary system. This is due in the main to the additives and colourings in our food which create an irritation. We know also that excess coffee drinking creates the same effect, and the brown dye in our cola drinks is lethal to the kidney and is said to be the reason for the high increase in kidney disease in persons of all ages today.

I remember the quite remarkable case of a man who had suffered agonies for years with renal colic and then kidney stones. He came to me for treatment, and as I worked upon his right foot he experienced great sensitivity in the kidney region. He explained that the kidney stones had been in the right kidney and it was quite obvious that the repeated episodes of kidney stones had caused erosions, which accounted for the sensitivity he felt. The following day he telephoned me and told me that later in the evening after my treatment session he felt sudden sharp pains again in his right kidney and then passed a large stone with very little discomfort, apart from some obvious localized bleeding. He was amazed and kept the stone to show me. Every time he had a treatment session he passed a small stone later the same evening, and this happened at least eight times until he was completely freed from his problems. He still comes to me occasionally for a general treatment.

# 11  The endocrine system

The endocrine system consists of the pineal, pituitary, hypo-thalamus, thyroid, parathyroid, thymus, adrenal gland, pancreas and the reproductive system. The endocrine glands are ductless structures whose secretions (hormones) pass directly into the circulation. All body cells require hormones, just as cells require nutrients. Hormones influence the activity of specific target tissues elsewhere in the body. There is a distinct and generally harmonious relationship between the various endocrine elements, whether they are separate organs (for example, the thyroid and parathyroids) or secretory cells lodged in other glands (for example, the Islets of Langerhans in the pancreas).

Control of the thyroid adrenal cortex and gonads is created by the pituitary gland. The hypothalmic gland has a controlling influence in growth, sexual activity, thyroid function, lactation, water balance, carbohydrate, protein and fat metabolism.

Release of adrenalin and noradrenalin places the body in the best possible condition for fight or flight reactions in addition to having direct effects on the heart, lungs and skeletal muscle. The blood sugar level is also increased in order to provide extra fuel for burning. You can therefore understand how anxiety and stress can cause physical disease. Excessive pituitary stimulation induced by higher nervous centres over a long period can result in damage to the cardiovascular system.

The parathyroids are small, usually four in number and, although embedded in the posterior aspect of the thyroid gland, have a function different from that of the thyroid in regulating plasma calcium and phosphorus levels.

The pituitary gland is situated between the eyes and behind the nose and is protected by an arch of bone called the Turkish saddle. The pituitary is often referred to as the master gland of the body, or the conductor of the orchestra. It produces seven distinct hormones: growth hormone (GH), controlling pre-pubertal development, adrenocorticotrophic hormone (ACTH), which affects the adrenal cortex; thyrotrophin (TSH)

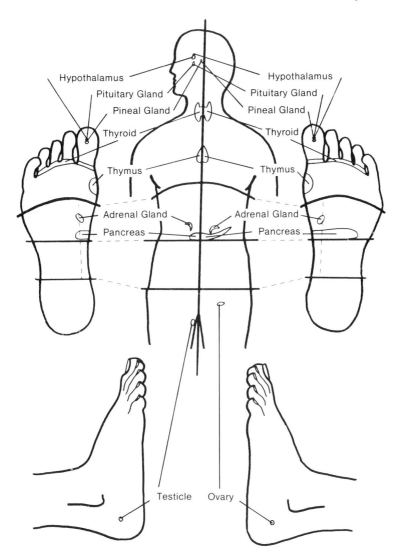

*Figure 7   The endocrine system*

to stimulate thyroid activity; prolactin (LTH), which activates the lacteal systems of the breast in pregnancy; follicle (FSH) and interstitial cell stimulating hormones (ICSH) controlling the reproductive system; and melanocyte (MSH) stimulating the hormone which affects skin pigmentation.

You can now appreciate the value of this amazing gland, which is only the size of a pea. It is therefore very important to work on this pituitary area for every single condition that you treat. It is to be found in the middle of each big toe.

The thyroid gland weighs about 28 g and is situated in the neck. It produces thyroxine. A baby born without a thyroid gland will be severely retarded because intellect does not develop without thyroxine. One of the vital constituents of thyroxine is body-building iodine. A deficiency in infancy or early childhood causes cretinism. In older people iodine deficiency causes hair loss, slowed speech and drying and thickening of the skin. Thyroxine also controls temperature. If the thyroid gland is removed from a rat it will build a thicker and bigger nest. People with over-active thyroid glands feel the heat, while those with underactive glands feel the cold.

The thymus is situated directly below the thyroid and parathyroid glands. Very little is known about this mysterious gland, but recent evidence suggests that it helps the body to recognize and reject foreign substances, including bacteria and viruses.

The adrenal glands are really the body's alarm system. Each weighs about 7 g and sits above the kidneys in the abdomen. Although they are anatomically linked, the adrenal glands serve different masters. They are comprised of the cortex and medulla. The medulla is an agent of the sympathetic nervous system and is therefore activated by nerve impulses. The cortex is an endocrine gland triggered by ACTH which is sent out from the pituitary. The adrenal gland helps the body cope with inflammatory conditions and is part of the body's reaction to stress, one of the major afflictions of modern life.

The pancreas gland, the sugar regulator in the body, is a large area of tissue lying behind the lower part of the stomach. It is the second largest gland in the body and takes its name from two

Greek words meaning 'all meat'. Without the effective working of the pancreas, food cannot be digested properly. The pancreas secretes two hormones into the blood, glucagon and insulin, produced respectively by alpha and beta cells in special areas of tissue called the Islets of Langerhans. Insulin, from the Latin word for 'island', is so named because it originates from these Islets. Diabetes occurs when the pancreas fails to secrete enough insulin and so fails to control sugar or glucose levels in the blood. Without insulin glucose accumulates in the blood. If glucose overflows into the urine, for example, it takes body water with it, resulting in acute thirst, which is one of the first signs of diabetes. Alternatively, starved of glucose, cells may start to burn up fat instead, causing weight loss. If insulin deficiency is serious and prolonged the diabetic sinks into a coma.

One of the most dramatically successful hormone treatments is insulin derived from pigs and cattle. It is estimated that the lives of some 25 million diabetics have been saved since two Canadians, Frederick G. Banting and Charles Best, extracted insulin from the pancreas during the early 1920s. Unfortunately, being a protein insulin is inactivated in the mouth, so has to be injected in carefully measured amounts.

Reflexology can help diabetic patients, but the very first question that we should ask from anybody seeking relief by this therapy is 'How long have you had the diabetes'. We can give relief to those patients who had a late onset diabetes – that is, a diabetic state which occurred in their mid-forties, perhaps after a sudden shock or severe infectious illness. However, it is difficult to offer much help to young children who have obviously been born with a defective pancreatic gland. The greatest benefit that our patients obtain is relief from the circulatory conditions to which they are liable. We know that diabetics are prone to heart conditions and problems with circulation in their legs in particular and that their healing processes are very poor, so here is where reflexology can give great help and relief.

It is necessary to work the whole of the digestive system when treating diabetics as well as to give a general and thorough treatment to all the other reflex points in the feet – which is a golden rule when treating, regardless of the condition for which the patient comes to you.

I have treated many diabetics during my career as a reflexologist. Some have been able to reduce their insulin intake, which is all to the good; others have experienced an improvement in their circulation and have generally felt fitter and have noticed an improvement in the healing processes of the body.

Virtually every cell in the body is affected by the hormones produced by the reproductive organs. The importance of the role these hormones play is felt throughout the human life-cycle. Sex hormones influence the reproductive capacities, maintain sexual urge and influence mental vigour and physical development. The reproductive organs produce hormones used by the adrenal glands and vice versa. This relationship may account for the effect the reproductive organs have in helping the body cope with allergies.

# 12 The central nervous system, spine and brain

The central nervous system consists of the brain and the spinal cord, with the spinal cord acting as the nerve link between the brain and the rest of the body. Motor pathways, as they are known, which carry impulses from the brain to the various organs of the body, descend through the spinal cord, while sensory pathways from the skin and other organs ascend through the spinal cord carrying messages to the brain.

The spinal cord weighs only 42 g, yet all limb movement depends upon it. About 43 cm long and 2 cm thick, it lies within the neural canal of the vertebral column. Nerves spring from the spinal cord, each pair serving a specific part of the body. Therefore, if the cord is injured, it is possible to detect which part is affected by examining functions in various parts of the body.

The spinal nerves are part of the peripheral nervous system, which also includes the autonomic nervous sytem and the cranial nerves. The skull is supported by the spine. The spine or spinal column which contains the tail and extension of the brain is built up of 26 vertebrae. Each vertebra is linked to the one above and below by joints and by flat, biscuit-shaped discs of cartilage, a flexible white tissue or gristle. These discs act as shock absorbers, softening the impact of jolts on the spine and allowing it to bend and rotate.

There are seven vertebrae in the neck or cervical region, the head being supported by the top vertebrae. Next come 12 thoracic vertebrae which support the ribs; the five lumbar vertebrae coincide with the small of the back; and at the base of the spine is the sacrum and coccyx or tail, a vestigial reminder of our past. The coccyx is the only bone in the human body without a function. The lumbar region of the spine receives the most wear and tear because of our upright posture, and consequently it is the seat of much back pain.

Reflexology gives immense relief to all spinal problems,

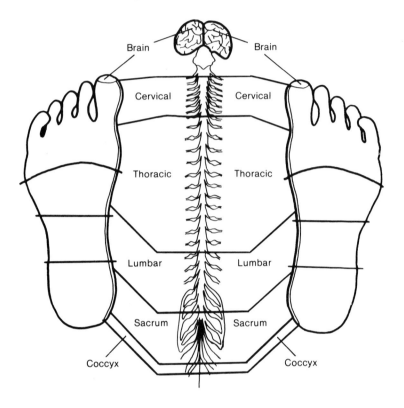

*Figure 8   The central nervous system, spine and brain*

particularly lumbago, sciatica, tension in the disc areas and pain caused as the result of a road accident or by sports injuries (see Figure 9). As there are almost epidemic proportions of back pain you will, in your experience as a therapist, find that a very large percentage of the patients that you treat are suffering back pain, and the results are very rewarding. I really cannot isolate one particular case that I have treated who benefited immensely because hundreds of patients have come to me hardly able to walk suffering from a back condition and in just a very few treatments have recovered their mobility and lost their pain.

The human nervous system is the outcome of millions of years of evolution. Man's predominance in the order of living

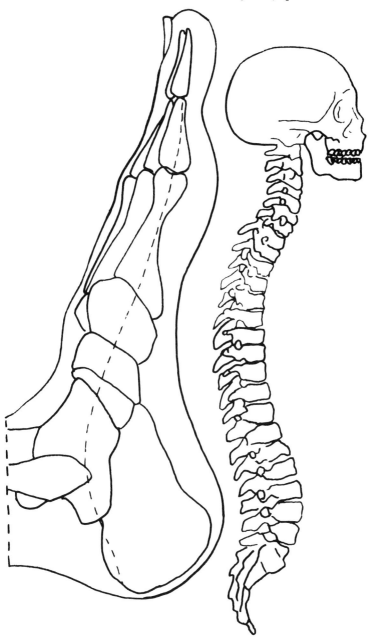

Note how accurately the shape of the foot relates to the curvature of the spine

*Figure 9   Spinal areas*

species is due entirely to the complexity and versatility of this system which, although deeply investigated by researchers, is still poorly understood. Its structure and activities are inseparable from every aspect of our daily lives, whether physical, intellectual or cultural. The millions upon millions of cells intermesh via a myriad connecting pathways to provide functions varying from the appreciation of literature to the fury of war. Despite recent huge advances in technology the brain is still the most versatile computer known to man, yet its vast complexity requires less power to run than a small electric light bulb. The nervous system has two responsibilities: maintenance of structural integrity by homeostatic control of the internal environment and adaptation to changing external circumstances. All living organisms exhibit these qualities to a lesser degree but the human nervous system has refined them to an unparalleled pitch.

Examination of the brain shows three distinct divisions which have structural counterparts in the story of vertebrate evolution. Ascending from the spinal cord and contained entirely within the rigid protective box of the skull are the hindbrain, midbrain and forebrain. Twelve pairs of cranial nerves are directly continuous with the brain.

Many of the diseases that affect the central nervous system will obtain some relief with reflexology, but only relief. I have treated patients suffering from multiple sclerosis and Parkinson's disease and they have received some relief, but I would say that these conditions show only a very minimal improvement. However, as there is very little alternative offered, it certainly is well worth working extensively on the areas related to the brain and spine, as well as thoroughly working out all the reflex points on both feet, just to see what benefit you get. With these demyelinating diseases it is essential to treat patients over a long period, at least one treatment a week for three months before any noticeable improvement will be seen.

I am particularly interested in the benefits that can be obtained in cases of brain-damaged children and have treated several in my years as a therapist. One little boy, in particular, remains in my memory and probably always will. Simon suffered brain damage as the result of a severe and unusual infection which damaged his brain cells. He went into a coma when he was eighteen months old and was not expected to live. However, he did eventually come out of the coma but was blind and unable to move. There was little hope medically and, as I knew the family, in desperation this little boy was brought to me. He did not move at all when treated; in fact, he was just like a breathing vegetable. I treated him weekly for months and months and, very very slowly, a little movement returned in his legs, then his trunk and arms. After six months of constant treatment he was able to sit, to recognize voices and began to utter a few words.

The hospital in London where he was a patient were amazed and keen to learn about reflexology. I was actually asked to send them a book on the subject, which I did. We continued treatment for a further year, and eventually he was able to walk with some support. Unfortunately Simon never recovered his sight and, when he was older, he went to a school for the blind.

You can never do any harm in trying to help somebody no matter how severe or 'hopeless' the situation may seem, and you will probably be pleasantly surprised at the wonders that can be achieved.

# 13   The lymphatic system

The blood carries oxygen and nutrients to the cells and waste products like carbon dioxide from them. However, not all the plasma (blood fluid) involved in these exchanges is reabsorbed into the circulation. That which is left behind in the space between the cells is removed by the lymphatic system, along with substances which are too big to squeeze through the capillary walls into the bloodstream. These include cell debris, fat globules and tiny protein particles. Once in the lymphatic system and mixed with plasma these are known as lymph. Thus the lymphatic system is the secondary transport system and the means of draining the intercellular spaces. The lymphatic system is also part of the body's defence system.

Excess fluid and other cargo is absorbed into lymph vessels, which are similar to blood vessels and lined with one-way valves, like veins, to prevent back-flow. Small lymph vessels join adjacent ones to form larger channels which lead to the neck where they empty into large veins.

Most of the lymph is eventually channelled into the 40 cm long thoracic duct on the left-hand side of the body. Every day the lymphatic system restores to the blood some 60 per cent of its plasma volume and approximately 50 per cent of the total amount of protein lost from the capillaries.

Lymph nodes are found at certain strategic points along the medium-sized lymph vessels: at the knee, elbow, armpit, groin, abdomen and chest. Acting as filters to trap bacteria and other debris, lymph nodes vary greatly in size. Swollen lymph glands may be felt in the armpit of a person with an infected hand or in the neck of somebody with infected tonsils.

Lymph vessels serve as carriers for cancer cells. For example, cells emanating from a malignant breast growth will travel along lymphatic vessels and multiply in the armpit lymph node. The node will enlarge and cease to function normally, enabling successive cancer cells to bypass it and affect other nodes in the lymphatic chain. This is why lymph nodes receiving lymph

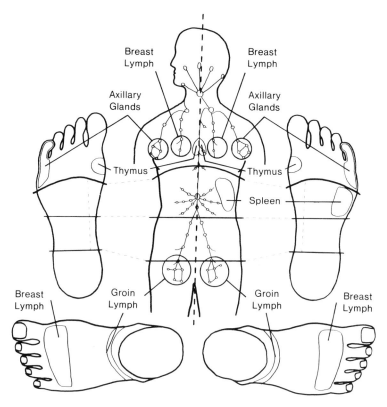

*Figure 10   The lymphatic system*

vessels issuing from a tumour are often removed along with the tumour. Unfortunately, it is not always possible to remove all the affected nodes.

Lymphocytes, a type of white blood cell, are packed in the lymph nodes. Lymphocytes produce antibodies, proteins which rise up against invading proteins known as antigens. The spleen and the thymus gland are also part of the lymphatic system. The spleen is involved in the removal of the blood cells and bacteria from the blood. Except for this all its other functions can be carried on by other organs, although children who have no spleens may have less immunity to bacterial infection than other children.

Overlying the heart the thymus consists largely of developing lymphocytes. After puberty it begins to shrink in size. Its role in the early years of life is not fully understood, but it appears necessary for the normal development of immunity.

The spleen lies between the bottom of the stomach and the diaphragm, and in a healthy child should be about 8 cm long and weigh no more than 98 g. In children or adults who have suffered repeated episodes of blood-borne infection – malaria, for example – it enlarges to huge proportions.

In actuality even the largest lymph nodes are only 2.5 cm across. Each node has several incoming lymph vessels but usually only one outgoing vessel and its inner structure is vaguely lobular. As in the kidney, the core of the node is known as the medulla and the outer part the cortex. The analogy is apt because a lymph node, like a kidney, provides an intricate network of spaces through which fluid is slowly filtered, its noxious contents being destroyed and its valuable contents recycled.

I have treated many patients, over the last years, who had suffered cancer in the breast and undergone a mastectomy. When a mastectomy takes place many of the lymph glands in the armpit are taken also and the patient usually suffers from fluid retention in the arm and shoulder area, with associated pain and stiffness. By treating the entire lymphatic areas, with much emphasis on working out the reflex point for the spleen, great relief has been obtained, and I can thoroughly recommend reflexology for this particular condition.

I remember treating a young Indian who suffered from repeated bouts of malaria. The only relief he ever got from the feverish symptoms was by having a daily reflexology treatment. This instantly reduced his temperature and relieved the aches and pains, and he was able to carry on with his life again.

# 14 The circulation

The continued existence of the many cells which make up human tissues is dependent on an adequate circulation. This provides the oxygen essential for metabolic processes and also removes the carbon dioxide formed as a waste product. The cardiovascular system is hydraulic since the transport medium is blood. A mechanical double pump (the heart) pulses the fluid at high pressure through a series of tubes (arteries and arterioles) which become smaller until virtually cell-size (capillaries). A collecting system of lower pressure (venules and veins) then returns de-oxygenated blood for a separate circulation via the right side of the heart and through the lungs. With oxygen content restored and carbon dioxide levels reduced by loss in expired air, the blood begins the whole circuit once again. The capillaries act as exchange vessels.

Where inflammation occurs the defensive (white) phagocytic cells can also cross the barrier. The residual pressure at this level also helps in the formation of lymph fluid within tissue spaces. This is eventually returned, after passing through the lymphatic system, to the right side of the heart. The amount of blood returning to the heart must be carefully controlled. The output of both left and right sides, despite the huge pressure differences between the systemic and pulmonary circulations, must remain the same, and there is a direct relationship between venous return and cardiac output.

The blood which returns from the stomach and intestine and also the pancreas and spleen is returned directly to the liver instead of the right side of the heart.

The heart is basically a hollow muscular organ weighing about 300 g. It is divided into four chambers and covered by two layers of pericardium. The heart does actually beat 36 million times a year. No self-contained substitute for the heart has yet been invented which can stand the hostile environment of the body and pump tons of blood around the body. Generations of poets and writers have earmarked the heart –

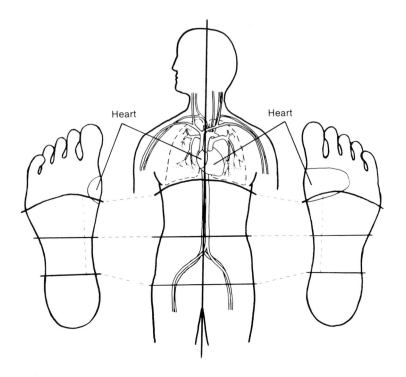

Heart · Heart

*Figure 11   The circulatory system*

which after all has no power over feelings for this special treatment in preference to the brain – the source of all thoughts and actions.

Coronary heart disease is the number one killer in industrialized countries. Sadly, it is a disease of affluence and technological progress. We exercise less today than at any other time in history. We no longer have to chase prey or run from predators. Instead, in our modern society, we save our legs at the expense of our hearts by using escalators, cars and other labour-saving devices.

Exercise strengthens muscle and thereby strengthens the heart. The heart beats on average 70 times per minute 100,000 times a day, 36 million times a year, and some 9,100 litres of blood pass through the heart per day.

The heart is approximately the size of its owner's fist. The top of the heart is level with the angle of the breastbone, one-third lying to the right of it and the rest to the left.

Much can be done in helping the body's circulatory system by using reflexology. If one concentrates on working out the entire heart and lung areas in both feet you will be able to relieve the pain of angina, and I have found great success in treating those patients who have suffered heart attacks. I remember treating a young man who had suffered a heart attack one month previously. He came to me in a breathless, exhausted state. After one month of having just two treatments a week his breathlessness disappeared and he was able to walk half a mile quite briskly without any undue effect. He went on having treatment for many months and made a remarkable recovery. He still attends for his monthly 'maintenance', as he calls it, and has been coming to me for years now.

High blood pressure is another serious threat to health. Each time the heart beats the arteries momentarily expand in proportion to the force of blood being pumped through them. This expansion can be felt when the pulse is taken. Blood pressure in the arteries is high but in the veins it is much lower. Hypertension is often called the 'silent killer' because it tends to be unaccompanied by any warning signs. Complications can cause kidney failure, coronary heart disease and strokes.

Fainting is a sign of temporary decrease in blood flow to the brain. The blood pools in the legs, reducing the flow to the heart, which in turn reduces the flow from the heart to the brain. Blood flow can be inhibited if one stands still for any length of time. Usually it can be restored to normal by very small movements, even toe wriggling or shifting to the other foot, but prolonged immobility – for example, when soldiers stand on parade – can cause a faint.

Once again, a good general reflexology treatment will lower the levels of high blood pressure. Special attention should be given to working on the kidney reflex area as the kidneys are always under a strain in this condition.

Remember, reflexology is not only to be used in helping the sick become well, it is invaluable in helping to maintain health.

# 15   The head, ear, nose and throat

In the struggle for survival that characterizes evolution the animals best able to employ natural environmental phenomena for hunting or hiding were the ones that survived. The ability to smell predator or prey, to hear noise and identify it with danger, or to use shade as a refuge were all features that helped in the never-ending conflict. Some evolutionary advances in the development of the special sense organs were critical for man's survival.

In man, the physiological functions of sight, smell, taste, hearing and touch all provide a central sensory input from highly sensitive receptor cells located in the eyes, nose, tongue, ears and skin. The electromagnetic radiation presenting as light in the visible spectrum is detected by the photoreceptors of the retina. To make this basic process more efficient, light energy is focused by a crystalline lens on to the retinal surface. The number of cells and their rich central connections allow a recognizable picture to be formed of the outsize world in which shape and form can be recognized, as well as movement. As evolution progressed, the location of the eyes changed from a lateral to a more anterior position. This meant that the visual fields overlapped to give binocular vision.

For efficient transmission of light the cornea must be kept clean and warm. These requirements are met by the constant secretion of tear fluid by the lachrymal glands. This is swept over the surface of the eye by blinking movements of the eyelids before collecting in the ducts. Here it drains and passes down the nose.

Man has a less well-developed sense of smell than many animals, and we know that infections of the sinuses can not only cause extreme pain and sensitivity to the upper part of the face and forehead but it can also cause a loss of both taste and smell.

Reflexology therefore is very beneficial in treating conditions of the eye such as glaucoma, frequent bouts of conjunctivitis and tired, strained eyes. Many people have exclaimed that they

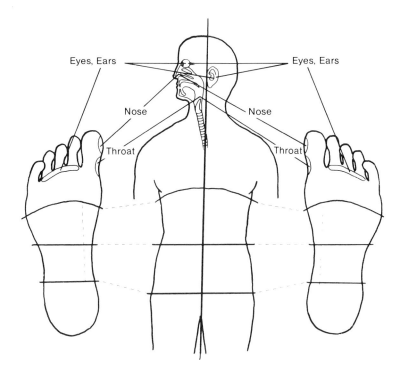

*Figure 12    The eyes, ears, nose and throat*

felt sure that their eyesight improved while having treatment for a sinus or eye condition.

As we work out all the toes on both feet we are working the sinus, eye, ear and nose areas. These will be extremely sensitive in those patients suffering from any of the above conditions.

The ear controls both hearing and balance. It consists of three parts, outer, middle and inner. The outer ear is the visible flap which we call our ear. It is divided from the middle ear by a passage lined with stiff hairs at the outer end to keep out foreign particles. It also contains glandular cells which produce wax, the purpose of which is to protect the ear from invading insects. This passage leads to the ear drum, which responds to high-pitched sounds by vibrating faster and to low-pitched sounds by vibrating more slowly.

These vibrations are transmitted to the amplifying system of

75

the middle ear. The human ear is not really designed to withstand prolonged high-intensity, man-made noise. It takes 36 hours to regain normal hearing after 100 minutes of non-stop exposure to excessive noise.

Ringing in the ear, or what is medically referred to as tinnitus, is quite a common condition today and can be greatly helped by treatment. Another very painful condition which occurs frequently in young children is inner ear infection. Here again, we can bring about great relief by working on the sinus, ear, nose and throat areas in the feet. As the ear, nose and throat are so closely linked it is quite common for bacteria which have settled in the throat or tonsil area to invade the eustachian tube and develop as a chronic ear condition.

The throat consists of a vertical muscular tubular structure which extends from the base of the skull and is divided into three parts. It contains two large lymphatic glands, the tonsils and also the larynx. The larynx has two groups of muscles, extrinsic muscles for overall movement as in swallowing, and intrinsic muscles which open and close the glottis during respiration, close the glottis in swallowing and regulate tension of the vocal chords for production of sound. The trachea or windpipe is a tubular structure of smooth muscle located in front of the oesophagus and supported by 16 to 20 C-shaped cartilage rings. It extends downward from the larynx (at the level of the sixth cervical vertebra) into the thorax, and then divides into two branches, the right and left bronchi, leading to the lungs.

Children in particular are prone to infections in the tonsil area. Regular treatment with reflexology can certainly help the infection and also, in many cases, has stopped the problem recurring.

# 16   The solar plexus

The solar plexus has a root in its Latin word that means 'to braid'. Anatomically a nerve plexus indicates a network or a group of nerve fibres intertwined and very elaborately interlaced with one another.

The solar plexus is a very large nerve plexus located behind the stomach and is often referred to as 'the abdominal brain'. The stomach is located in the left side of the body. The solar plexus is composed of two large ganglia from which many smaller ones in semi-lunar or crescent shapes are distributed to many places.

There are about ten subdivisions. The ganglion is a mass of nerve tissue containing nerve cells. The ganglion is like a little energy centre placed outside of the brain and the spinal cord. Both of the solar plexus ganglia are prevertebral, which means that they are located outside of the spinal column.

The sympathetic nervous system is therefore a part, a subdivision, of the solar plexus. According to its functions the sympathetic nervous system is also a division of the part of the human nervous system which is called the autonomic nervous system. It controls and monitors the involuntary functions of the human organs. These functions are performed automatically and independently of our will. They cannot be consciously controlled.

The solar plexus along with the sympathetic nervous system, which again is a subdivision of the solar plexus, controls the marvellously orchestrated sequential events in our system, upon which our lives depend. The solar plexus presides over the sympathetic nervous system, and it is said that it is fully developed and already performing vital functions in the early stages of the human embryo – at a time when even the human brain is not fully developed.

Thus we see that the solar plexus is the greatest nerve centre. It presides over most of the autonomic nervous system. It even organizes the blood circulation by changing the volume of

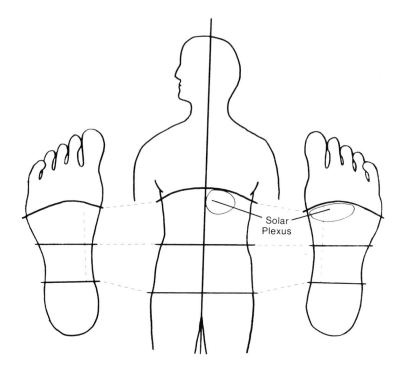

*Figure 13    The solar plexus*

blood that passes through the blood vessels. It regulates the circulation of vital forces and electromagnetic impulses flowing through the system. Therefore the solar plexus is also the source of vital force and physical energy and the great storehouse thereof, as well as being its generator. It actually has solar (sunlike) qualities.

It is also referred to as a 'feeling brain'. It is a centre of feeling and emotions. One can experience a very special sensation in and below the chest when a strong emotion arises. People often describe it as 'being sick to the stomach', but it is really a sensation in the solar plexus. Every mental and physical state has a physical manifestation. It is a well-known fact that an injury to the solar plexus disturbs the natural life processes, and a strong blow to this area can even cause instantaneous death.

In order to obtain the best results in reflexology, the

maximum benefit to be obtained will be by working on the left foot. By working out the entire diaphragm/solar plexus first on the left and then on the right great relaxation will be experienced. It is therefore of great importance to commence a treatment session by working out this area and repeat the process at regular intervals throughout the treatment session, as it is the most vital area in obtaining both mental and physical relaxation.

# 17   You – the reflexologist

Whether you intend using reflexology as a profession or only to help your friends and family is irrelevant. What you must do is to learn to master the science with accuracy. There are certain disciplines that are essential to follow. When you introduce anyone to the benefits and principles of reflexology your level of self-confidence and self-discipline in what you say or do will have a significant effect on the initial reaction of the patient. Obviously, you will meet many sceptics along your pathway, as reflexology is still somewhat untraditional by nature.

Be sure you know exactly what reflexology is:

It is a science that deals with the principle that there are reflexes in the feet relative to each and every organ function and part of the human body.

Be sure you know what it does:

Reflexology relaxes tension, it improves nerve and blood supply and restores balance to the body.

Reflexology can never harm. It is therefore not dangerous to treat young children or the very elderly. It *is* safe to treat pregnant women; in fact, they receive much relief from the discomforts of pregnancy, swollen feet, digestive upsets, backache and so on. We cannot use reflexology to diagnose specific diseases, but the feet will tell us that an organ, function or part is in a congested, sluggish or tense state, and by working on the reflexes in the feet that reflect this condition by their very sensitivity we are able to encourage an improvement in the functioning of the body.

Don't promise any 'cures' or offer a 'course of treatments'. People can vary on just how long it takes for them to receive an improvement in their health. Many do have instant relief, and this can happen even if the problem has been with them for years. In fact, it is quite incredible to hear, 'I have been suffering from this problem for years, have seen several specialists, have taken all manner of drugs and have had several episodes of pain and disability. Just one visit to you and I feel a new person.' It really is amazing.

You will also treat the patient with a very minor condition who makes many visits before an improvement is shown.

Do present a professional image – a grubby, untidy room will give the impression of a non-caring person. The room in which you treat your patients should be pleasantly decorated with a comfortable massage couch or reclining chair. Make sure there are plenty of pillows available to make your patient comfortable. Use a spotlessly clean large towel to cover your patient's legs when you are giving a treatment.

Take the trouble to have some pleasant relaxing music playing in the background, and a few nice plants or pictures will all add to the 'caring' you offer.

Now, what about your hands! They are going to be on show. Your hands and nails should be well cared for, and, in particular, your nails should be short and well filed. This is essential otherwise your patient will feel the discomfort of your nails on his or her foot.

Hold the foot firmly, with authority and using a firm, controlled pressure work through the foot with tiny, tiny forward-creeping movements of the thumb, in particular. The index finger can also, on occasions, be used.

Use the relaxation techniques at the beginning and end of a treatment session and during the progress of treatment. These you will be taught during your training as a reflexologist. Observe your patient's expression. If she or he flinches, reduce the pressure. Reflexology can cause discomfort, at times, particularly if there have been years and years of a build-up of congestion in the body through the use of drugs, but a treatment should never cause 'extreme pain'. If it does then the therapist has been badly trained.

Remember, our whole aim is to relax tension. If we inflict too much pain the patient will instantly 'tense up' and the whole principle of the science will be destroyed.

As you work through the feet of your patient he or she will ask you to explain what reflex you are working upon when experiencing sensitivity. The patient has a right to know, after all; it is his body that you are treating. Give a direct answer. I always explain that the sensitivity that is being experienced is related to the liver or kidney area or wherever it might be, and the reason for the discomfort is an indication that there is a lot of congestion and tension in that area, and is often caused as the result of medications, food additives or colourings or because the patient has had much infection in her body (if this is so).

It will take about 40 minutes to give a good treatment session (when you are experienced). In your early days as a new therapist it may take you the best part of one hour. Be sure to adhere to the 'Golden Rule', never, never, just treat one or two specific areas in the feet to help a specific area in the body. Always treat every section of the foot each time you give a treatment. Remember we are working on the holistic principle of treatment, and this means treating every reflex point in the foot every time. This will restore the body back to its maximum potential and create this general feeling of well-being.

If the patient who comes to you for help is in acute pain then I suggest you treat two or three times a week for the first week. By this time much of the pain should have reduced. Then go on to give a treatment on a weekly basis. If you are treating a general chronic state, most people respond well to a weekly session and have great relief in about six treatment sessions. If the patient feels much improved after, say, four visits to you, suggest that you leave the appointment for two weeks and just see how the situation is after a fortnight.

If the improvement has been maintained then suggest that the patient return to you in a month's time for a further appointment. If all is well after a month then it is a very good indication that the problem has been eliminated, and suggest to your patient that she contact you again in the future if the problem recurs.

You will find that many of your patients feel so fit and well after a treatment session that they prefer to see you for an occasional treatment to maintain their good health.

Your approach to people is a vital ingredient to your success as a therapist. You will, in time, learn how to be sympathetic when sympathy is needed, how to show compassion, and at other times it will be necessary to exhibit some firmness when patients allow minuscule problems to build in their minds as mountains.

Depressed patients can drain you, if you allow them to. When I meet people who are so low that life seems not worth living, and who hint at 'ending it all', I use a very good first-aid remedy. Give them a piece of paper and divide the page into two columns; then ask them to list the good things about themselves, and some beauty in the outside world. Depressed people have a very poor self-image, and I think a bed of roses would look like a heap of manure to a person suffering from this condition. When they return with the paper it will usually contain about five items of 'good' and fifty-five of bad.

I then help them to complete the paper on the 'positive' side. Remind them that behind that sad face is a person who used to paint, play tennis, enjoy good music, help her neighbour – and did she realize that she has lovely hair, a super complexion and a wonderful figure? This very simple therapy works as a 'mental tonic'; try it with one of your friends or family who are going through a bad passage in life.

You will also have to learn the ability to keep other people's problems at arm's length. It is impossible to solve the problems of the world, and if you go to bed at night worrying yourself about everybody's problems you will soon be far sicker than those you treat.

Remember, your body is your total responsibility. It belongs to nobody else, and it is not the responsibility of anybody on God's earth to 'heal' anybody of anything. Your body was built with the wonderful ability to heal itself, once put into the right 'atmosphere'. We as therapists can only act as channels for this wonderful energy, and if a patient fails to respond to you or your treatment, don't take it as a personal rejection. Perhaps you could advise him or her to try another form of complementary medicine. This has on quite a few occasions happened to me, and I always get in touch with the patient later on to see if the herbalism, homeopathy or whatever it was they sought was helpful. You should feel joyous when they are well, not slighted. What we should be looking for is freedom from pain and suffering for the patient, no matter who achieves the success. Healing should never be used as a boost to the ego of the therapist!

There should never be any need to advertise your services. A good therapist will find that his or her greatest advertisement will be the satisfied people who have been under their care. Patients will talk about the wonderful relief they obtained from treatment with reflexology, and news will soon spread. After all, what is the most usual greeting between two people? 'Hello. How are you?'

# Conclusion

Apart from the basic information and historical evidence contained in this book, which I hope will stimulate the appetite of those who are becoming increasingly aware of the growth of alternative medicine – in particular, reflexology – I sincerely hope that those of you who will go on to study and become professional reflexologists will experience the interest and joy I have had in treating the general public these last full ten years.

I have actually given some 12,000 reflexology treatment sessions, apart from the many hundreds of therapists I have trained. I could write another book just on the people I have met and helped and the happy and heart-rending experiences that I have encountered.

The most incredible fact about illness is that it can happen to any one of us, no matter what our colour, race or creed. Whether we have abundant riches or dire poverty is irrelevant, as neither state offers us the solution to disease.

I have treated sick people from all walks of life. They have come to me in their chauffeur-driven Rolls-Royces with their long, sad, tense faces, uptight with their business problems, their life styles, their families, and worried sick on how to manage their fortunes. I have yet to meet a very wealthy person who is at peace with himself.

Then there are the local country folk who come with their aches and pains. They often cycle or walk, as they are unable to afford to run a car. Many of them have brought me a bag of produce grown in their own gardens because money is very short and they are unable to find sufficient for a treatment; their appreciation is shown by a gift which is gratefully accepted. I always say to my students, and will repeat it again. If you turn people away because they are unable to find sufficient money for a treatment, then you should not be working as a therapist. There must be some fundamental basis of humility to want to help people at all. There are certain qualities, other than qualification, that make a nurse a 'special' nurse, and there are definitely certain qualities needed in becoming a reflexologist other than passing your examination. You need to be able to offer a consistent, reliable service to the public. People get used to knowing the days and times that you work and know that you will always be available to give of your best.

Reflexology is a very 'private therapy' and there are only ever two people involved, you and your patient. As the years go by you will treat families who involve you in all the events in their lives – the births, deaths and marriages. In fact I have just started treating the children of many young teenagers whom I helped some ten years ago. It is wonderful to feel that they have sufficient confidence still in the benefits they received for themselves that ten years later they are bringing their young children to me for treatment.

I regularly receive a yearly postcard from a young boy I treated nine years ago for his chronic asthmatic state. He had spent the best part of his early years in hospital. When he was 12 his parents brought him to me for treatment and he had a very rapid response to reflexology. In fact, his asthma disappeared altogether, and within six months he was as fit as a fiddle, able to play sports for the first time in his life. He grew big and strong and became so fit that he joined an athletics team. He proved his potential there and was eventually chosen to run in the Olympics. His yearly card sings the praises of reflexology and the treatment, he says, that 'changed his life'.

I get a great thrill in training those who have no medical background or experience whatsoever, but who feel that a career in the field of healing is something to which they are drawn. It certainly does not mean that those with a medical qualification in some other science make the best therapists.

I find, in general, that those people who have had a wonderful result from reflexology and are therefore utterly convinced of its benefits have a great enthusiasm to study and practise and go on to make excellent therapists. Some of my most successful therapists were those who knew nothing about alternative medicine or orthodox medicine whatsoever, but were fired with a desire to learn.

If you feel that you have had a long-standing disorder that

does not seem to have been relieved by orthodox medical treatments, then give reflexology a try. It can never do you any harm, and in 95 per cent of cases it does such a lot of good – but don't expect an instant miracle. It took you time to become ill; it will take a little time to get well again.

I can honestly say that I have never once in my career in this rewarding work ever felt bored, or not looked upon each day as one which would bring me in touch with more people who I could 'convert' to the true benefits of reflexology, and I have never given a lecture where I have not failed to interest even the most sceptical regarding the virtues and benefits to be obtained from this treatment which I so genuinely and passionately believe in.

I once read a book on reflexology which changed the whole direction of the rest of my life. Maybe reading this will have the same effect upon yours!

# Index

Page numbers in italic refer to figures in the text.

# Index